Also by the Authors

Aromatherapy for Scentual Awareness
Aromatherapy for Lovers and Dreamers
Aromatherapy for Scents and Sensuality

Aromatherapy for *Men*

KAREN DOWNES

AND

JUDITH WHITE

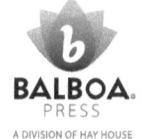

BALBOA.
PRESS

A DIVISION OF HAY HOUSE

Copyright © 2011 Karen Downes and Judith White

The moral right of the authors has been asserted.

All rights reserved. No part of this book may be used or reproduced by any means, graphic, electronic, or mechanical, including photocopying, recording, taping or by any information storage retrieval system without the written permission of the publisher except in the case of brief quotations embodied in critical articles and reviews.

Balboa Press books may be ordered through booksellers or by contacting:

Balboa Press
A Division of Hay House
1663 Liberty Drive
Bloomington, IN 47403
www.balboapress.com
1-(877) 407-4847

Because of the dynamic nature of the Internet, any web addresses or links contained in this book may have changed since publication and may no longer be valid. The views expressed in this work are solely those of the author and do not necessarily reflect the views of the publisher, and the publisher hereby disclaims any responsibility for them.

ISBN: 978-1-4525-0205-2 (sc)
ISBN: 978-1-4525-0209-0 (e)

Any people depicted in stock imagery provided by Thinkstock are models, and such images are being used for illustrative purposes only. Certain stock imagery © Thinkstock.

Printed in the United States of America

Balboa Press rev. date: 6/6/2011

Front Cover Photo by Bobbi Fabian
Editing by Shanna Provost

*This book is dedicated to all
the men in our lives, especially those
who have inspired us to write these words.*

Acknowledgements

We would like to thank Shanna Provost for the many hours she has put into researching and editing this book. Katerina Lettas for overseeing the whole project and keeping us on track. Finally, our buddy and fellow adventurer, Leon Nacson.

Contents

Introduction

OUR AROMATHERAPY WORKSHOPS HAVE ALWAYS been popular with women, but we've noticed an increasing number of men attending in the last two years or so. No, they haven't lost a bet and they haven't always been dragged in by well-meaning girlfriends and wives! They come of their own accord and are always willing to plunge head-first into the aromatic world of essential oils.

We've also found ourselves speaking to an increasing number of men at business conferences and meetings as the male-dominated corporate industry catches on to what has been known for centuries: essential oils are powerful tools that can be easily enjoyed by men and women. For example, in the workplace they can help reduce stress and increase self-esteem, creativity and productivity.

It seems to be a sign of the times that gender roles are becoming less defined as equality of the sexes comes into balance. Women are filtering into previously male-dominated areas, feeling more confident, discovering new ways to express themselves and focusing on their career paths. Men are becoming more interested in grooming and nurturing themselves and are discovering the importance of being able to express their inner thoughts and emotions.

Many men are going beyond the 'shower, shampoo, shave' approach to personal care and are looking for ways to make the most of what they've been given. In their busy lives they know that in order to stay on track and remain focused they have to feel good about themselves. Essential oils are perfect vehicles to this end, as they work effectively on many different levels and purvey natural aromas which appeal to everyone.

Not only are men finding aromatherapy valuable for self-improvement, they have also realised that their women love it, especially when the oils are lovingly applied through a relaxing massage. And many men have found that the right combination of oils applied in the right places can be very enticing. Since ancient times, pharaohs have indulged their bodies, warriors have prepared for battle and emperors have delighted their senses with essential oil combinations.

As aromatherapy is a *wholistic* modality, it works on the whole person. In fact, so powerful are essential oils that they possess anti-viral and anti-bacterial properties, working actively on the body whilst rejuvenating the spirit with healing vapours.

In our experience, men are happiest when they are achieving more than one thing at a time, and that's exactly what happens when essential oils are used properly. Not only can the physical appearance be enhanced, but self-esteem and self-confidence can also improve. As men begin to look better, they also begin to feel better about themselves, because the essential oils work to uplift and revitalise the body, mind and emotions.

It is important that we all, male and female, acknowledge our self worth and learn to nurture ourselves. While it's nice to have others to care for us, it's also important to strike a balance between being cared for and being the carer.

The softer, more nurturing qualities within us all can be brought out beautifully while the power and strength of our bodies can be revitalised with aromatherapy. In modern society aggression and domination are no longer effective tools for moving life forward and attaining goals. Today's ambitions are about developing that inner power, expressing that unique identity and putting it all into action.

We don't have individual aromatherapy courses for men and women in our *Aromatic Health Care* programs because aromatherapy addresses life, and in this book you will discover an aromatherapy lifestyle you can live and breathe regardless of your sex. Because a man's regime is quite different to that of a woman's, we will discuss how men can use essential oils most effectively and suggest blends for improving appearance, health and overall wellbeing.

So, gentlemen, if you want to look and feel great, you've come to the right place! So too have you women who are looking for gentle, affirming ways to help your man adapt more easily to these changing modern times.

— *Karen and Judith*

1

Scents for Success

THE BASICS OF AROMATHERAPY

"HE WOULD NOW STUDY PERFUMES AND THE
SECRETS OF THEIR MANUFACTURE, DISTILLING
HEAVILY SCENTED GUMS FROM THE EAST."

Oscar Wilde, The *Picture of Dorian Gray*

AROMATHERAPY, AS THE TERM SUGGESTS, IS based on a healing technique which uses the aromas provided by Mother Nature in plants, trees and flowers. These aromatic substances are called essential oils and are taken from various botanical species around the world that have been prized for their wonderful healing properties since time began. Today, we know it is both the *aroma* as well as the *chemical makeup* of an essential oil that supports our health and wellbeing. Scientists have proven through olfactory research that the aromatic molecules of essential oils permeate the nasal mucosa and reach the limbic part of the brain where memory exists and emotions are triggered.

Each essential oil is composed of 150-200 naturally occurring chemical constituents which produce a chemical reaction in the body. For example, all essential oils have anti-bacterial properties to a lesser or greater degree.

Historically, essential oils have been used for trade, religious ceremonies and healing. Whilst our knowledge of their healing powers has certainly developed dramatically since those ancient times, the way in which we use them and the benefits we derive from them are not too dissimilar to those of our ancestors. We still celebrate the benefit and delight that oils bring into our lives today.

Our ancestors knew exactly what they were doing when they prepared their bodies for lovemaking; they used aromatic balms to soothe the heart and calm the emotions and restored their battle-weary bodies in aromatic baths. Their secrets have been passed down from generation to generation, and with our modern-day technology we can validate scientifically what our forefathers knew intuitively. Chemists around the world are testing devices, the most common being a *Gas Chromatograph* which tests the chemical composition of an essential oil. Through this analysis we know the components that will be entering the body and what action they will perform.

The power of the oils lies not just within their anti-bacterial healing properties, but also in their ability to instantaneously bring about change to feelings and emotions. The chemical complexity of essential oils has been graciously created by Mother Nature and it is the naturally occurring chemicals (primarily for the plant's protection and procreation) that makes every essential oil unique in its quality and function.

There are two main ways in which essential oils enter the body: via the hair follicles of the skin and through the olfactory system, the nose. So you can now discover ways in which to embrace aromatherapy as an everyday part of your life, to arouse your sensual awareness while at the same time contributing to your health and vitality.

The Sense of Smell

Many men believe the words they use have the most profound effect on creating or projecting an image. In our highly-developed society, our sensory acuity is so finely tuned that the impact we make on others occurs well before we open our mouths to speak. We make our sensory decisions about each other a few seconds after we meet. Deep friendship and romantic alliances are dependent upon what scientists identify as 'olfactory bonding'. Studies show that fragrances make a considerable impact on social relationships. A study done by Drs John Neziek and Glen Shean (College of William and Mary Fragrance and Social Behaviour), sponsored by the Fragrance Research Fund, showed that when people believed their fragrance was pleasing to others they felt more confident in their social interaction. Scientists have proven that it is our sense of smell which is responsible for attraction or repulsion from others.

The odiferous molecules are picked up by the nasal *mucosa* and transported via a nerve pathway to the brain where it registers within four seconds. Imagine being able to alter the way you think and feel in such a short amount of time simply by breathing!

Our subconscious mind receives and responds to a scent way before our conscious mind has time to think about it. Odours and scents act as powerful stimuli in a part of the brain which is responsible for governing the major glands in our body. These glands, in turn, are responsible for our emotional and even our sexual responses to others. You will have already discovered how odours provoke an immediate response. Have you ever smelt a loved one's article of clothing or a familiar perfume and felt immediately connected to that person? Odour is also closely linked to our memory, but we'll go into that in more detail in Chapter 5. There is no other sense that is such an open portal to the outside environment.

Stop for a moment and think about how you project your identity every day. Is it with an identifiable aftershave filled with aromatic chemicals and alcohol, or could it be that every morning you take two minutes to create your own personal signature scent for that particular day out of natural oils? You could be carried into your day with a home-made decoction of aromatic oils that you have designed to stimulate, entice and intoxicate the senses with subtlety, mystery and allure.

Feel Your Way

Some people attempt to cover or disguise their true body scent whilst others consider it a natural part of their makeup. No two people will interpret a fragrance in exactly the same way. Our sense of smell is exactly like our personal fingerprint. Keeping this in mind, use your intuition and creativity to create your own signature blend each and every morning.

Although the temptation will be there, don't become too regimented and disciplined in the selection of your essential oils by always basing your choice on their function or purpose. It's better to take a moment to consider what you have ahead of you in your day and choose your oils using your *senses* to select those aromas that will support you in the tasks ahead. Perhaps you need greater focus with *Lemon* oil, or a sense of inspiration from those tall and magnificent pine trees. Often your intuition or sense of smell will guide you.

And so it is when choosing an oil blend for another. You must check in with your senses before applying the oil to your body. Can you imagine sitting down to a plate of food that you dislike the smell of, or that your body rejects, and thinking that it will be good for you? Most unlikely! Once you have created your mix, simply ask the recipient if your creation pleases their senses or if they find it offensive in any way.

Provided the person does not strongly object to the smell, it will be fine to apply it. In our experience, whilst most people are accustomed to using perfumes, sometimes their initial response to the smell of oils will simply require an adjustment to smelling something that is totally natural.

After using oils for some time, you will find that your sense of smell becomes more finely-tuned and your sensory perceptions to your outside environment will be more acute - a fantastic skill to have in this rapidly changing world.

2

Laying the Foundations

ESSENTIAL OILS AND
THEIR APPLICATIONS

"THAT WHICH WE CALL A ROSE BY ANY
OTHER WORD WOULD SMELL AS SWEET."

William Shakespeare, *Romeo and Juliet*

YOU WILL NEED SOME BASIC TOOLS TO BEGIN to practise the art
of aromatherapy. Also, it will help if you familiarise yourself
with a few terms that are mentioned often throughout this
book. Don't worry if this is unfamiliar ground to you, it will
soon begin to make sense as you delve deeper into the world
of aromatherapy.

Utensils You Will Need

I.   100ml In Essence Aromatherapy Blending Bottle (amber
     or cobalt blue glass).

2. Two aromatherapy vaporisers: one for home and one for use at work.

3. Vaporiser candles (small, round candles the size of a 20 cent piece that burn for 9 hours).

4. Small glass mixing bowl three inches (75mm) in diameter.

5. A selection of high quality pure essential oils (up to 40).

6. Massage base oils (*Sweet Almond* or *Jojoba*).

Terms You Need To Know

ESSENTIAL OIL

A fragrant, volatile liquid extracted by means of distillation or expression from a single, botanical source.

BLENDING BOTTLE

When blending your aromatic combinations of oils or mixing a massage oil for yourself or others, you will require some empty glass bottles as described above. The coloured bottles work much better than clear glass bottles because they keep the light from reacting with the oils.

BLENDING BOWL

This can be a small glass or ceramic (never plastic) bowl approximately three inches in diameter in which to mix your daily massage blend. Oils can dissolve the 'filler' in certain plastics, which, in turn, can adulterate your essential oil blend. If you use plastic, make sure it is impervious to essential oils.

MASSAGE BASE OILS

Cold-pressed vegetable oils are used as a massage base oil to carry essential oils over the body. They are usually high in vitamins and nutrients to nourish the skin. The two base oils are *Jojoba (a natural fluid wax)* and *Sweet Almond*. It's a good idea to keep them in the refrigerator until just before use to keep them fresh, especially in warmer climates.

VAPORISER

The ideal way to vaporise (allow the aroma to permeate a room via an aromatic vaporised mist) essential oils is to use a ceramic vaporiser. Vaporisers are available at most leading department and specialty stores. Eight drops in total of the chosen oil (or a combination of oils) are placed in the shallow dish at the top of the unit that has been filled with warm water. A *vaporiser* candle - which can last up to nine hours - is lit underneath the dish. The heat from the candle gently evaporates the water and oils together into the surrounding atmosphere, allowing you to enjoy their healing vapours.

The A-Z of Essential Oils

Now it's time to get to know the essential oils and their healing properties. This will help you choose the right blend for yourself or someone else. The oils we have included in our aromatic selection give you versatility, whether you are looking for a medicinal aid or an improvement to the way your skin looks and feels.

BASIL
Country of origin: Egypt

AN uplifting oil which has a clarifying effect on the brain. You can use *Basil* for concentration and decision making and as a compress to relieve mental fatigue.

An ideal choice if you're just about to conduct or attend a business conference, or for any environment where you are wanting the participants to be more focused when receiving important data that is to be remembered. If you're studying, call on *Basil* to assist you to focus your concentration.

Basil assists in the treatment of all kinds of respiratory ailments such as bronchitis. To relieve a migraine headache simply dispense one drop of *Basil* onto one of your middle fingers, press both middle fingers together so that you have a little *Basil* oil on each finger, then massage the neat oil onto your temples and onto the base of your skull above your spine. A compress will also help relieve a migraine. *Basil* is also an excellent nerve tonic.

Basil oil, pale yellow in colour, is distilled from the leaves of the *Basil* plant.

Caution: *Avoid topically during pregnancy.*

BERGAMOT
Country of origin: Calabria, Italy

BERGAMOT is a very uplifting oil. It helps to disperse nervous anxiety or depression and relieves nervous tension. Its fragrance invites you to feel relief from the burden of the tasks at hand. If you are a teacher, presenter or facilitator of information to an audience, simply breathe in the aromatic vapours to disperse those pre-presentation jitters. A lawyer told us that he now puts a drop on his handkerchief and discretely breathes in (he pretends to blow his nose) before he speaks to a jury.

A versatile oil with many uses, its fragrance blends well with other oils. As a massage oil it is excellent when treating acne and oily skin problems or dermatitis.

This delightfully fresh and citrus essential oil is made by pressing the rind of a fruit like a miniature orange. *Bergamot* is the distinct flavour found in Earl Grey Tea.

Caution: *Photosensitive: Do not use externally in the presence of ultra violet light, ie: when sunbathing or using sun beds.*

BLACK PEPPER
Country of origin: India

THIS oil brings comfort and direction to those needing to make changes in their life. Endurance and motivation are two potent qualities of this activating oil.

Use *Black Pepper* to ease away muscular aches and pains or stiffness after physical exertion. This essential oil assists to strengthen poor muscle tone and revive the body from fatigue.

An excellent oil to use for enhancing your self-image, building your self-esteem and instilling a greater sense of confidence when facing the boss or the board. A great oil for those long days at the office when patience wears thin and your energy levels flag.

CARDAMON
Country of origin: Central America

FORTITUDE and courage are attributes of this spicy oil. This is an oil for those times when you feel stretched, as it relieves mental fatigue and nervous strain, bringing purpose and inspiration. It is also said to possess aphrodisiac qualities.

A great oil to relieve indigestion and flatulence when massaged on to the digestive tract and abdominal area. Brings comfort to heartburn and colic.

A great addition to an aftershave lotion. As an oil to remedy stress, it will revive your body and mind, so soak in an aromatic *Cardamon* bath at the end of the day or blend with a floral oil such as *Rose* or exotic *Jasmine Absolute* for a romantic interlude.

CEDARWOOD
Country of origin: USA

ONE of the oldest known essential oils, *Cedarwood* may be used to release chronic anxiety and reduce stress. It is often used in men's toiletries. Through the ages, pharaohs, emperors and lords have been entombed or buried in Cedar coffins.

The fragrance of *Cedarwood* brings emotional support and balance to the tasks at hand. Whether they be personal or work-related issues, you can count on *Cedarwood* to restore the peace. If you have any conflict between work colleagues or with teenage children expressing their desire for independence, you can call on *Cedarwood* to provide a more harmonious atmosphere.

Cedarwood used in a vaporiser or inhaled is a great help with chest complaints such as catarrh and bronchitis. Used in conjunction with *Rosemary*, it can assist in restoring hair growth and can retard thinning hair. Genuine Cedarwood essential oil comes from the wood of *Junipers Virginiana* grown in the USA and is related to the biblical 'Cedar of Lebanon'. Its fragrance is that of the freshly-cut tree.

CHAMOMILE

(ROMAN & GERMAN)

Countries of origin: England and Germany

THESE two varieties of *Chamomile* are similar. They can calm and soothe the savage beast within. Because they affect both the body and mind, you can use them to treat inflammation.

Roman Chamomile is a particularly sweet fragrance compared to *German Chamomile* which is far more herbaceous. *Roman Chamomile* goes well in social situations such as cocktail or dinner parties, children's parties or family gatherings. It is effective when seeking relief from wind in the gut, as in the case of colic. *German Chamomile* is most useful when specific relief is required, whether it be physical or emotional, as it has wonderful anti-inflammatory properties.

It can be used in the treatment of skin allergies such as eczema or to ease the symptoms of red, inflamed skin. A handy oil to use in a massage blend or vaporiser to release yourself from emotional rage. *Chamomile* is often used with children, and both varieties have long been part of herbal medicine. Their properties work exceptionally well with *Lavender*.

CLARY SAGE
Country of origin: Austria

THIS oil is the most euphoric of all essential oils. It is particularly effective in the type of stress-related problems many people experience. It helps to relax and uplift the most despondent person and release depressed thinking.

This is definitely a 'feeling great' fragrance which can be used to enhance any business lunch. *Clary Sage* is the essential oil to wear when you plan to 'party', go out on the town or simply put yourself into a 'peak' state.

It can be used as a compress and in a massage blend for general relaxation. The woman in your life can relieve her menstrual pains by making up a small massage blend and applying it to the abdominal area.

Distilled in the northern hemisphere from the *Clary Sage* flowers, it has a sharp and slightly nutty aroma.

Caution: *Avoid topically during pregnancy.*

CYPRESS
Country of origin: Spain

HELPS to disperse nervous tension, especially if you feel that you're being pulled in a number of directions. *Cypress* seems to help create order amongst chaos.

Call on *Cypress* when you are preparing budgets, forecasts or reports and any time that you want to be more focused and centered.

Cypress may help to prevent asthma attacks and treat whooping cough and croup. It is also useful in treating conditions where excess fluid is a problem. It is ideal as an aftershave splash if you have oily skin.

This highly astringent oil is distilled from the leaves and berries of the tree. Its woody fragrance is often used in men's toiletries.

EUCALYPTUS
Countries of origin: Australia and China

EUCALYPTUS oil has a cleansing and energising effect on the mind and body and a deodorising effect on the environment. It is the best-known protection for winter ills. The anti-viral qualities of *Eucalyptus* can protect you when you share a house or office with others who have colds or to clear the air in your temporary home when you are travelling.

If you work out, use it in a massage blend after exercising. It will reduce or eliminate the lactic acid build-up in muscle tissue which is the cause of muscular discomfort after exercise. *Eucalyptus* can bring relief to arthritic pain.

Eucalyptus is an excellent decongestant and its anti-bacterial and anti-viral properties can help to stop the spread of infections. You can use it to relieve the pain and itching of chicken pox, shingles and cold sores. Some surgeons use *Eucalyptus*-impregnated gauze to cover wounds.

There are many species of gum tree in Australia, and in aromatherapy the leaves from *Eucalyptus Globulus* are distilled to make one of the many *Eucalyptus* oils.

Caution: *Avoid topically during pregnancy.*

FENNEL
Country of origin: Spain

IDEAL as an alternative to *Peppermint, Fennel* aids the digestive system because it relieves nausea, colic and flatulence and is the ideal after-dinner 'mint'.

If you enjoy eating lots of spicy foods, especially those hot curries that make you cry, indigestion can be the unpleasant aftermath. Simply make up a *Fennel* massage blend and rub it over your stomach before you go dining and again when you come home to help eliminate that gastric reflux.

The oil is distilled from the dried and crushed seeds of the Mediterranean plant which has a delicious aniseed aroma.

Caution: *Avoid topically during pregnancy. Avoid topically on hypersensitive or damaged skin.*

FRANKINCENSE
Country of origin: East Africa

THE effect of *Frankincense* on the mind and emotions is calming and it may be used to promote a quietening of the mind when meditating or to help unwind after an overwhelming day. This oil is excellent for dispersing fear, to fortify and to comfort.

When you are getting ready to present a new proposal, requesting a raise in salary, going before a review board or if you have to front someone after you have made a huge 'faux pas', then this is the oil to call on as it disperses that momentary fear or paranoia.

Frankincense has a rejuvenating effect and is especially good for mature skin. If you and your skin spend a lot of time outdoors, add a few drops into your morning body rub.

The resin from which *Frankincense* is distilled has been burnt on altars for centuries. It has a penetrating, soothing aroma.

Caution: *Do not apply to hypersensitive or damaged skin.*

GERANIUM
Country of origin: Egypt

A GOOD balancer for mood swings or emotional highs and lows during those 'mid-life' experiences and through times of change. It has a calming and relaxing effect if you're feeling uptight. When you're out there performing in a busy career as well as trying to balance the demands of a relationship and family, your emotions can feel like they are on a rollercoaster ride. This is the time for *Geranium*, the restorer of balance.

Geranium has uses in skin care, particularly when the skin is dry, as with dermatitis, eczema and severe cases of dandruff. Very good in the bath or as a hair rinse.

The distilled leaves produce a typical 'flower' oil used regularly in the perfumery industry as a substitute for *Rose*. It is a balancing and harmonising oil which originates mainly from North Africa.

Caution: *Not to be used topically on red and inflamed skin.*

GINGER
Country of origin: China

WITH its warming qualities, *Ginger* is a great booster of confidence. It energises and strengthens the body and the mind.

Wherever rigidity occurs in the body, be it arthritis, muscular stiffness and tension or even in the case of poor circulation, this oil gets things moving. If you love to ski, give yourself another warm, protective layer to brave the cold. Add *Ginger* to your morning body rub!

Use *Ginger* to rebuild and re-energise your body if you are showing signs of debilitation at the end of a stressful week. Use it in a vaporiser at work to keep a project moving and at the same time to keep you on the project.

Caution: *Avoid topically during pregnancy.*

GRAPEFRUIT
Country of origin: East Mediterranean

UPLIFTING and refreshing, this is an oil that alleviates stress and anxiety. It promotes alertness and sharpens the senses for greater performance.

Grapefruit is a valuable oil for protection against infectious diseases when used in a massage blend. Use it to energise and activate the body before exercise.

It's a good oil to use for new experiences and to promote spontaneity and co-operation in others, especially when entertaining and celebrating. If you want to inspire new ideas, add several drops to your vaporiser.

Caution: *Photosensitive: Do not use externally in the presence of ultra violet light, ie: when sunbathing or using sun beds.*

Jasmine Absolute
Country of origin: India

An extremely sensual extract which arouses and warms. It restores a deep sense of confidence and elevates self-esteem. *Jasmine Absolute* is an excellent oil to bring balance and optimism, most helpful when choosing to release frigidity (either emotional or physical) or depression.

This oil is renowned for its aphrodisiac qualities and ability to arouse physically and emotionally. It can be used to soften dry, irritated and sensitive skins.

It has been used to alleviate nervous exhaustion and for people with difficulty in communicating, to bring sensitivity and openness to the conversation. This is definitely an oil to use to restore romance and sensuality to your relationship, especially if you've put in long hours at the office and your partner needs some nurturing.

JUNIPER
Country of origin: Austria

JUNIPER works on the emotions to rid the mind of 'waste', thereby relieving anxiety. As a purifier of the blood, it can be used to relieve the symptoms of arthritis, joint pain and gout. People who play a lot of sport, especially tennis or golf, can greatly benefit their joints by adding Juniper to their body rubs.

If you have been consuming lots of alcohol you will benefit from a *Juniper, Lemongrass* and *Rose* body rub. One man, when purchasing a bottle of *Rose* just to make up this recipe, said: "I'm paying for this hangover in more ways than one." We believe he was referring to the price of *Rose* oil.

Juniper can be used for the relief of fluid retention and other toxic wastes such as those connected with acne. (Please note: *Juniper* is not a diuretic).

The Chinese revere the tree for its immortal quality. The oil is distilled from its ripe berries and has a fresh aroma like turpentine. *Juniper* is an ingredient of gin and works to stimulate the appetite - hence the drink 'gin and tonic' as an aperitif.

LAVENDER
Country of origin: Bulgaria

PROBABLY the most popular and versatile essential oil, *Lavender* has a soothing and calming effect, balancing and normalising any given condition.

Its properties range from anti-bacterial and cell stimulating to acting as a sedative and insect repellent. It may be used in a vaporiser, inhaled or applied neat, with a cotton bud on unbroken skin, or in dilution, depending on the treatment required.

If you're feeling irritable, agitated, short tempered or finding that you are taking everything personally, especially as a result of working long hours, travelling or recovering from being ill, then call on *Lavender* to soothe away those frayed emotions. Wearing *Lavender* is nearly as nurturing as having a pair of loving arms draped around your neck and a soothing word whispered into your ear.

A highly active or sleepless child can often be calmed with a few drops of *Lavender* on the pillow. It's an excellent oil as a general tonic when you're recovering from an illness. It can be strengthening and nurturing.

LEMON
Country of origin: Sicily

AN excellent tonic, particularly to refresh and uplift, *Lemon* oil helps the body defend against infection. A wonderful oil to enliven any environment, especially when you return home after the house has been locked up for a while. Open the windows and let *Lemon* loose.

When you want to stay wide awake and enlivened whilst reading, reviewing or studying, call on *Lemon* essential oil as it stimulates focus during study and relieves the mind from brain strain. In or out of the office, this is a refreshing clean fragrance that switches focus on and distraction off.

Used neat in combination with *Thyme* essential oil, it can get rid of warts. It is useful for treatment with oily skin. Just add one drop to your facial moisturiser (see Chapter 3).

This essential oil is pressed from the outer rind of the fruit and has the familiar citrus aroma.

Caution: *Photosensitive: Do not use externally in the presence of ultra violet light, ie: when sunbathing or using sun beds.*

LEMONGRASS
Country of origin: India

LEMONGRASS oil is tonifying and cleansing for the whole body. It is a fortifying oil which may help modify nervous tension.

Recover from intense physical activity - such as a day working in the garden, building or renovating, a long hard workout at the gym, or being up all night with your lover - in a *Lemongrass* bath. This oil will revive the weariest man.

This traditional Chinese and Indian medicinal plant has a powerful tonic and stimulating effect on the whole system. The leaves, from which the essential oil is distilled, are often used in cooking.

Caution: *Avoid topically during pregnancy. Avoid topically on hypersensitive or damaged skin.*

LIME
Country of origin: Peru

LIME, along with the rest of the citrus family, is refreshing and uplifting. This oil promotes clarity and assertiveness, making it an excellent choice if you're feeling doubt or confusion.

By actively working on clearing physical as well as emotional issues, this oil is great for obesity, congestion and poor circulation. It helps to clear problem or blemished skin when diluted into a massage base oil.

Use in your morning body rub-down in preparation for a board meeting where a clear head and focused thoughts are needed or when making decisions about new directions or changes in your life. (See Chapter 3). Because of its stimulating effect on circulation, you can use *Lime* oil to induce warmth to cold hands and feet or to move you into activity. Just add a few drops to a carrier oil and rub the blend on the hands and feet.

Caution: *Do not use externally in the presence of ultraviolet light, ie: sunbathing or sunbeds.*

MANDARIN
Country of origin: Sicily

THE mandarin's sweetness inspires and brings a sense of calm and tranquillity. This oil is a favourite for restlessness and insomnia as it soothes away anxiety and tension.

Mandarin is excellent for digestive disorders and intestinal discomfort, especially when massaged onto the abdominal area in a clockwise direction. It helps to move excess fluid in the body and activates the liver.

Use *Mandarin* for aromatic bathing before retiring for a restful sleep or to add zest to an aromatic aftershave.

Caution: *Do not use externally in the presence of ultraviolet light, ie: sunbathing or sunbeds.*

MARJORAM
Country of origin: Egypt

THE warm, penetrating aroma of *Marjoram* works to lessen both physical and emotional responses. Its comforting properties help those experiencing grief.

It is excellent in a massage base oil for hurt muscles and tension. *Marjoram* works well as a sedative in a warm bath and blends well with *Lavender.* This is the oil to choose when your body and soul are crying out for deep relaxation.

Marjoram, as an excellent sleep inducer, will help to rebalance the body's 'time clock' for shift workers.

Caution: *Avoid topically during pregnancy.*

Myrrh
Country of origin: East Africa

Myrrh is strengthening and rejuvenating. This is the oil to use when you are heading out into the physical or emotional marathons of life. When you really want support, know that *Myrrh* will come to the party, especially when you have to pull out all the stops physically, mentally and emotionally to meet deadlines.

This thick, sticky, reddish brown oil has a pungent aroma and is a very good expectorant and astringent, helping with all kinds of coughs and colds. As a first aid, use one drop of *Myrrh* on a cotton bud and apply it to heal mouth ulcers. It can also be used in the treatment of gum disorders by adding one drop of *Myrrh* to your toothpaste before brushing.

This rare oil is distilled from the resin of a small, thorny tree which grows in difficult countryside. Legend has it that Arab shepherds collected the resin from the beards of their goats.

NEROLI

Country of origin: Tunisia

ESPECIALLY helpful when you want to minimise anxiety, it can bring relief to all kinds of stressful situations. When you reduce stress and anxiety, you increase your sensual arousal. Sensuality is of the body and senses as distinct from the intellect. It can only rise when you leave the problem solving of the world to someone else for a while.

Neroli makes you feel more settled, especially if you are tossing and turning prior to sleep. It calms hysterical behaviour and is an excellent vein tonic. If you have varicose veins or broken capillaries (red cheeks or nose is the visual display for broken capillaries) then use *Neroli* and reduce your salt and alcohol intake and your exposure to extremes in temperature.

Because *Neroli* assists new cell growth, it is useful in skin care, particularly for dry skin.

This oil takes its name from an Italian princess who used it as her favourite perfume. Distilled from the flowers of the Seville orange, it has a beautiful perfume, particularly when diluted.

ORANGE
Country of origin: Brazil

LOOKING for more fun, more enjoyment and celebration? Then call for *Orange*. Used in a vaporiser, *Orange* is excellent to set the mood for entertaining, especially when it's combined with *Bergamot*.

Orange is the perfect choice when you want to 'hang out', spend time with the boys or read the weekend papers. Use *Orange* oil in your vaporiser at work if you are wanting to inspire creativity in yourself or others. Brainstorming sessions are assisted by this sweet fragrance which lures people into participation.

Orange relieves the restlessness of insomnia, creating an opening for rest, and can help ease acute headaches. In skin care it is useful for cleansing oily skin. If you smoke, try using *Orange* as a compress to soften and release any congested pores.

Distilled from the outer peel of oranges, this refreshing and uplifting oil blends well with others.

Caution: *Do not use externally in the presence of ultraviolet light, ie: sunbathing or sunbeds.*

PALMAROSA
Country of origin: India

WITH its ability to calm and strengthen, this oil is excellent for nervous exhaustion as it brings balance and restoration to frayed nerves.

Use in your daily skin care regime to prevent dryness after shaving (See Chapter 3). Add one drop to a small amount of *Jojoba* oil to assist the healing process. Use with *Lavender* to heal scar tissue. It can also be used for its antiseptic qualities to relieve the symptoms of colds and 'flu.

Use *Palmarosa* to quieten and calm any frantic thoughts or when your mind feels overactive. Add several drops to your vaporiser at the end of a busy day or in the office environment when all around seems to be in chaos.

PATCHOULI
Country of origin: Indonesia

THIS oil has a rich Eastern aroma which can relieve anxiety and depression and may even have an aphrodisiac quality, particularly when blended with *Ylang Ylang*. *Patchouli* really came into its own in the 1960s when it was used to promote love and peace as opposed to war.

It has a deep, provocative aroma and used as a body rub, can increase your masculine charm. If you have been feeling down in the dumps, draw on the uplifting qualities of *Patchouli*. You may choose to combine some of the citrus or floral fragrances from your other essential oils so that you modify the exotic perfume.

It works well as an antiseptic to heal chapped or broken skin and fungal infections including athlete's foot. Old scar tissue responds well to a blend of *Patchouli* and *Lavender*.

Peppermint
Country of origin: USA

As one of the stimulating essential oils, *Peppermint* promotes clear thinking, activates the brain and engages thoughts.

This is the ideal choice after lunch when the body and mind move into 'snooze time'. Just inhale the enlivening vapours and your mind clears while your body naturally engages in deep, slow breathing.

If your ears block when travelling by aircraft, simply put one drop of *Peppermint* onto a small piece of cotton wool and roll it between your fingers to spread the essential oil. Break the wool into two pieces and make two small ear plugs. Insert them just inside the ear to clear the ears and ease the discomfort.

The classic stomach/digestive remedy, *Peppermint* has excellent anti-spasmodic properties and is a pleasant general stimulant. Inhaled directly from the bottle, it clears the head and is an effective treatment for travel sickness or sinus congestion.

Caution: *Avoid topically during pregnancy. Those who suffer from epilepsy or convulsions should also avoid its use.*

PETITGRAIN
Country of origin: Paraguay

THIS oil brings an inner sense of strength and stability. With its fortifying qualities it encourages communication, expressiveness and openness.

A great hair tonic for oily or greasy scalps. In the summer months especially, *Petitgrain* makes an excellent anti-perspirant.

Use *Petitgrain* as a tonic for the nervous system whilst recovering from any stress-related conditions. Use it at the office in your vaporiser to expand your thinking and to be able to speak your thoughts more openly.

PINE
Country of origin: Siberia

INHALATIONS of *Pine* oil are good for relieving chest colds and catarrh. It also has a stimulating effect on the circulation. This essential oil is particularly good for adults who suffer from asthma or as a tonic to the lungs of those who smoke.

The pine needles are firm, strong and directional by nature. The pine tree in nature exudes strength and purpose and these are the qualities that your body drinks in as you absorb the aromatic molecules.

Pine can inspire you and provide you with purpose and direction which can be useful when you are at the crossroads in your life. This oil can support you through career and relationship changes.

Dry distillation of the needles, cones and young twigs collected in northern Europe and Russia produces a pale, fresh, resinous aroma.

Caution: *Avoid topically on hypersensitive or damaged skin.*

Rose
Country of origin: Bulgaria

THE most potent healer of the essential oils. Just one drop is all you'll require for most purposes. The exquisite and powerful perfume works on the depths of your emotions, nurturing and restoring power and confidence. Cleopatra made *Rose* oil famous for its aphrodisiac qualities.

You can use *Rose* essential oil for personal or professional indulgence. It can create potential and possibility from the most bizarre circumstances. On those days when you feel that staying in bed is the best option, use the essence of *Rose* oil to draw you back into action. It is the right choice when you want to let go of anger at yourself or others.

Rose works powerfully on your body, especially on the reproductive system and it has a restorative effect on the liver (especially after a generous drinking session). It is particularly valuable for use in skin care as a tonic.

One of the elite essential oils, it wears a price tag better regarded as a 'personal investment' as it takes thousands of rose petals from Bulgaria to make one drop of *Rose*.

Rosemary
Country of origin: Morocco

Rosemary has a strong effect on the nervous system, acting as a brain stimulant to heighten sensory perception and memory.

Some people believe that when it comes to taking in information, their brain functions like a funnel: the information goes in one ear and out the other. If you can relate to that analogy and you are frustrated by it, try *Rosemary* in your daily body rub or vaporiser.

Rosemary is the ultimate choice when you want to switch remembrance on and forgetfulness off. It is also a very good oil to use in massage, helping tired or injured muscles. Traditionally used in hair care, mostly as a rinse or scalp rub, it can stimulate hair regrowth.

One of the earliest used oils, *Rosemary* essential oil is distilled in Morocco, Yugoslavia, Spain and France.

Caution: *Avoid topically during pregnancy. Those who suffer from epilepsy or convulsions should also avoid its use.*

ROSEWOOD
Country of origin: Brazil

To emotionally rebalance and recharge, this oil carries a restorative quality both emotionally and physically and it elevates and uplifts even the most despondent mood.

A cleansing tonic for the body when used in massage, *Rosewood* carries antiseptic properties which promote the body's own natural defence system, thereby assisting in fighting coughs, colds and winter chills.

If you have been pushed to the extreme, soak in a *Rosewood* aromatic bath at the end of the day. Add it to your vaporiser at work to sustain your energy levels throughout the day.

This tropical evergreen tree with a reddish bark and heart-wood is native to the Amazon region. *Rosewood* blends well with most oils, especially citrus, woods and florals.

SAGE

Country of origin: Albania

A HIGHLY antiseptic oil, *Sage* can be used to cleanse the mind and skin. It has a fresh, clean fragrance that most men relate to. The fact that it is one of the most deodorising essential oils to the body makes it specifically suited to the active males.

Smelly feet and armpits surrender to the essence of Sage. This is the oil to cleanse the day away, especially if you intend to go out on the town with your partner. If you class yourself as a bit of a 'rager' and plan on dancing the night away, then prepare your body with an aromatic soak in *Sage*.

The deep-cleansing qualities of *Sage* help purify the dirtiest pores and skin. If you work in dust and grime or smoke, you will do well to compress your skin morning and evening with this oil. (See Chapter 3.)

Valued throughout time as a sacred herb, it sources mainly from south-eastern Europe.

Caution: *Avoid topically during pregnancy. Those who suffer from epilepsy or convulsions should also avoid its use.*

SANDALWOOD
Country of origin: India ~ Eastern District

A STRENGTHENING aroma which releases irrational fears, *Sandalwood* can have a stabilising influence through many life changes. It is used to promote strength and courage especially for people undergoing a lot of changes.

If endurance is the call of the moment then *Sandalwood* is your choice. The long meeting, hanging in there with your partner through childbirth, a long night making love, a hard workout at the gym - whatever the lengthy occasion, allow *Sandalwood* to contribute to your staying power.

As a cosmetic ingredient, *Sandalwood* brings moisture to dry skin as well as giving a pleasant aroma liked by both men and women. It has been used most successfully to treat sore throats and laryngitis.

The oil is distilled from the heart-wood of the tree. Long used in India as a perfume and incense, *Sandalwood* seems to live up to its reputation as an aphrodisiac.

TEA TREE
Country of origin: Australia

WELL known to Australians, *Tea Tree* oil has many uses and is unique in that it is active against bacteria, viruses and funguses. This is a must to have in your first aid pack at home, at work and play.

If there was ever first aid in a bottle, this is it. If you have a mouth ulcer, boil, infected cut or abrasion, gum disorder, tinea, wart, wasp or bee sting, thrush - whenever you need an antibacterial agent, *Tea Tree* is the oil to use.

It is also a powerful immune-stimulant which helps the body to respond by fighting invading organisms. This oil protects you when you wear it on your body. It has an energising effect on the body and mind, especially when used first thing in the morning. It is tonifying when used as a massage oil.

Caution: *Avoid topically during pregnancy.*

THYME
Country of origin: Spain

IF you liken *Tea Tree* to the soldier against bacteria, then it is appropriate to call *Thyme* the army.

This is a powerful force against long-term colds, 'flu or viruses that seem to persist. *Thyme* acts as an anti-oxidant in the body and therefore becomes an essential ingredient in morning body rubs. It is said to prolong the degeneration of brain cells in the elderly, thus being an element of anti-aging regimes in both men and women.

This is a potent oil and only the smallest amount is all that is required to produce results.

It is an excellent oil for respiratory, mouth and throat infections (never use directly inside the mouth, on the vagina or on any mucous membrane, as this oil is very strong), it works to stimulate the production of white blood cells to strengthen the body's resistance to infection.

Its refreshing herbaceous fragrance blends well with *Sandalwood*.

Caution: *Avoid topically during pregnancy. Avoid topically on hypersensitive or damaged skin. (A mucous membrane irritant).*

VETIVER
Country of origin: Java

A DEEPLY relaxing oil, *Vetiver* comes from the root of the plant and is responsible for its nourishment. We therefore acknowledge the drawing power of *Vetiver* as the bearer of opportunities and possibilities.

Vetiver has long been associated with success and abundance. It is a powerful ally when you are putting out for good fortune, whether it be related to a new job, career or financial situation. This is the perfect choice to include in your morning body rub if you are going into any negotiation.

It is valuable as a bath oil and for use in massage. It brings strength to the deeper layers of the skin and supports the body's ability to absorb nutrients. It is used successfully to alleviate stress and is a useful skin care aid for mature skin types.

YLANG YLANG
Country of origin: Comores Islands
(off the coast of North Africa)

A STRONGLY exotic sensual oil which blends well with other floral, citrussy and woody oils. An anti-depressant essence possessing sedative and aphrodisiac qualities, *Ylang Ylang* is mainly used for its calming and relaxing properties.

Ylang Ylang has the ability to arouse the senses. It has a provocative and alluring fragrance and is a tonic to the emotions of the heart. It helps disperse anger and frustration and is the perfect accompaniment to social situations.

It is most effective in your skin care program as it has a balancing effect on both dry and oily skins. It will help regulate rapid heart beat and rapid breathing.

Originating in Indonesia, *Ylang Ylang* is used in perfumery and cosmetics. The powerful aroma is from the 'flower of flowers' and is identifiably heavy and sweet.

Caution: *Not to be used topically on red and inflamed skin.*

NOTE

1. Essential oils should not be used undiluted over large areas of the body.

2. Avoid direct contact with the eyes.

3. Essential oils are not soluble in water. If irritation or allergic reaction occurs, remove immediately with a massage base oil or milk.

4. The quality of essential oils will vary according to climatic conditions and geographical location. This may alter from time to time and takes constant research and monitoring by aromatherapy suppliers to always maintain the best.

5. The countries of origin mentioned in this chapter are based on our most current research. Future developments in the essential oil industry may initiate the availability of high quality essential oils from other locations around the globe.

3

Polishing the Image

AROMATHERAPY FOR SKIN FITNESS

"I THINK THERE IS A FEMININE SIDE TO ALL
MEN, IT'S JUST THE RATIO THAT VARIES."

Andrew Olle

YOUR SKIN IS SIMPLY A REFLECTION OF YOUR internal mechanics coupled with the external environment: the sum of what you feed your body, how you care for it and what you subject it to. You may already know that the skin is the largest organ of the body and it must be nourished and cared for in order for it to function well.

Ultimately, your skin will always reveal to the world how you look after yourself.

While your whole appearance will certainly not go unnoticed, people pay attention to your face when they're talking to you. How you are caring for yourself on all levels will be mirrored to the outside world every day. If your face shows signs of stress and fatigue or a careless attitude towards grooming, that promotion, new job or business deal may well go to the man with the cleanest and brightest image.

A well cared for skin can also give men a more competitive edge in the workplace. Job interviews, presentations, meetings, conferences and business lunches are all times when the spotlight is on, and who wouldn't want to put their best face forward? This is something that you must apply yourself to in your everyday life if you want to achieve long-term positive results and not just a quick attempt at grooming in the moment.

For many years the basics of personal grooming for men have been adequate: making the effort to dry-clean your best suit, polish your shoes, cut your nails, comb your hair, brush your teeth and apply deodorant. But when it comes to their face, most men give it a quick wash with soap and water, shave it and splash it with an aftershave.

While many men can look more distinguished as they age, a lifetime of neglect will eventuate in a tired, wrinkled-looking skin which looks weary rather than worldly. A face that spells laziness could have adverse effects on both business and social dealings, not to mention the way men feel about themselves. The benefit of using essential oils is that they are an investment in your health on all levels, impacting on the way you think, feel and act.

How quickly do we look at another and automatically make an assessment about how they present themselves? What is it that you think when you see a man with an unshaven face and greyish or sallow-looking complexion? Probably the same as what we women think: this man doesn't care about himself. While the image of the rugged Aussie male is a stereotype which has long been held up as desirable, the truth is that most women would much rather get close to a smooth, clean face than a flaking, dehydrated skin covered with shaving spots and a rash.

Taking time and effort to look after your body in a new way doesn't mean denying your natural masculine characteristics. Many men are now trying to be more caring and sensitive for their women, developing their more intuitive side, and it is a continuing quest for them to strike a happy medium between being strong and supportive, yet vulnerable and open. We believe the answer lies in nurturing and valuing yourself while pursuing the development of your own potential.

You will find many techniques to look after both your own personal needs and to complement your partner's as these pages unfold.

In short, go for the best you can be! Enhance your enthusiasm and communication, increase your personal power and live the abundant lifestyle you richly deserve with the help of your new aromatherapy program.

The Skin Program

ESSENTIAL OILS FOR THE SKIN

Lavender, Bergamot, Cedarwood, Sandalwood, Cypress, Lemon, Rosewood, Mandarin, Juniper, Sage, Tea Tree, Ylang Ylang.

We recommend that you follow this program on a daily basis for the best results. For optimum skin fitness you must work on the inside *and* outside of your body to assist in elimination and regeneration. So don't forget to address your dietary needs for a healthy body.

We know that many of you will already be thinking, "Who has the time to do this?" If this is the case, stop and think again. These simple techniques are a short extension of your daily personal hygiene routine (and a more nurturing way of doing what you are already doing). A few extra tools coupled with your essential oils can start you working on all levels of your wellbeing today.

The time spent in this simple daily program is also affirming for your subconscious mind that you are worthy of this extra few minutes. The end result is that you will feel much better about yourself and the ultimate expression of this will show through a confident, self-assured persona, an energised body and an uplifted spirit.

Like any good businessman knows, when you are clever with your investment of time and money, you will reap generous rewards. Think about that body you will have for the rest of your life and what bonus you would like it to provide in years to come, then invest in it accordingly. But you'll need to begin today!

Aromatic Shower/Body Brushing

What a great way to start the day! Imagine stepping into the fresh smell of pine needles or the embracing aroma of a *Eucalypt* forest as these aromas permeate the shower vapours. Wet body brushing is a simple and natural process which stimulates your circulation and brings a healthy glow to your skin. At the same time it will assist in the elimination of waste products and the dead cells that can build up on your skin that make it look dull and sallow. Your body and mind will be stimulated into action.

Utensils: 100ml In Essence Aromatherapy Blending Bottle (amber or cobalt blue glass), your choice of oils, 1 natural-bristle body brush (available at chemists and department stores).

1. Fill the glass bottle with warm water.
2. Add 3-5 drops of your chosen oil or oils and shake vigorously. *(Go back to Chapter 2 to choose your oils)*.
3. If using soap, wash your body first then rinse off.
4. Standing out from under the running water, sprinkle your aromatic water all over your damp body.
5. Use the wet body brush to stimulate the skin, as if you were polishing a pair of shoes with a backward and forward action. Don't be too gentle, your skin is a sturdy organ. Polish your whole body.

Aromatic Dressing/Body Rub

Begin your day by creating an aromatic blend, choosing your essential oil combination based on the type of day you are anticipating (busy, demanding, creative). Standing in front of your selection of essential oils, choose your blend in much the same way you would decide what to wear, depending on the weather, the occasion, scheduled meetings etc. Remember, you are now dressing from the *inside* out. You are dressing your body with oil to protect and nourish its largest organ (the skin) and addressing your emotional needs before dressing with your outer garments. Your skin should be left feeling more alive, with a healthy glow to it. If it is greasy in any way, you have applied too much oil, so lightly towel off the excess. Remember next time to apply a small amount with each application and rub in briskly.

Utensils: 1 glass or ceramic blending bowl, your choice of oils, base massage oil, 1 measuring glass.

1. Measure 10mls of your massage base oil *(see base oils in Chapter 2)* into your blending bowl.
2. Add three to five drops in total of your chosen essential oils (it's best to combine no more than three oils at any given time).
3. Begin by dipping your fingers into the bowl and taking up a small amount of oil. Rub your hands together to disperse the oil evenly over the hands and, starting at your feet, smooth the oil over with a swift rubbing action, moving up the leg.
4. As the oil is rubbed in, dip into the bowl again and repeat the procedure, moving up and over the body.
5. The more hair you have on your body, the more oil you will need. You should feel like you are glowing at the

end of the rub but not feel greasy. You should be able to dress on completion. If you feel you need to towel excess oil off, you've used too much.

Pre-shave soak

Utensils: I clean flannel or face cloth, *Lavender* oil.

1. Fill the bathroom basin with warm to hot water.
2. Add a few drops of *Lavender* essential oil. Agitate the water to disperse the oil molecules.
3. Soak the flannel in the aromatic water and squeeze the excess water out. Leave the cloth damp.
4. Soften the skin by using a pressing and releasing action with the face cloth. You simply press the flannel into the skin then move to another part of the face. Move over the entire face and neck area. Do this three or four times before shaving. This cleanses the skin, opens the pores and prepares it for shaving.

Aftershave Splash

You will need any combination of three of the following oils:

Lavender, Bergamot, Tea Tree (as an antiseptic), Cedarwood, Sandalwood, Geranium, Cardamon, Black Pepper, Palmarosa.

100ml glass bottle

1. Add 2 drops each of *Lavender, Bergamot* and *Tea Tree* oil for example, to a blending bottle filled with 100mls of pure water.
2. Shake the bottle vigorously with the lid intact to disperse the oil through the water.

3. Splash a small amount of this blend on the face to tone and soothe the skin after shaving and prior to moisturising. Create your own favourite combinations.

Skin Regenerator/moisturiser

Shaving daily can be quite drying to the skin. This moisturising blend will quickly help to soften and regenerate, leaving you feeling revitalised.

1. Blend 1 drop of *Lavender* with 1ml of *Jojoba* oil and smooth it onto the skin. *(Soothes and settles the skin after shaving and softens regrowth.)*
2. For a more 'earthy' blend, use 1 drop of *Cedarwood* with 1ml *Jojoba* oil. *(Regenerates and softens the skin after shaving.)*
3. If you're on the go and don't have time to use this program, simply continue your body rub blend as listed earlier.

The Evening Cleanse

It's important to cleanse and tone as per the pre-shave soak every evening before retiring (see *Pre-Shave Soak* method in this chapter). The soaking procedure prepares you for sleep, removing the dirt and grime of the day and softening the skin to prepare it for overnight regeneration. This soaking can be done with many essential oils. We recommend the following selections:

Grapefruit — 2 drops or	*Rosewood — 2 drops*
Geranium — 2 drops	*Lavender — 2 drops*
Sandalwood — 2 drops	*Black Pepper — 2 drops*

Cardamon – 2 drops or	*Lavender – 2 drops*
Palmarosa – 2 drops	*Bergamot – 2 drops*
Frankincense – 2 drops	*Cedarwood – 2 drops*

FOR THE FEET

Foot odour dusting powder

Sage – 2 drops	*Tea Tree – 1 drop*

1 tablespoon baking powder

This oil combination can also be used in a footbath.

Acne

Acne can be more of a problem for men than women, especially when shaving, but the correct use of essential oils can help dramatically as all essential oils are antiseptic to a lesser or greater degree, depending on the essential oil.

Acne can occur on the face, the neck, back and chest. It manifests as blackheads and spots, sometimes with scarring, pitting and inflammation. The temptation to squeeze the spots and remove the infected pus may be great, but you should refrain from this as it can cause scarring.

Acne is often the result of poor dietary and lifestyle habits. This leads to a hormonal imbalance and a condition known as *seborrhoea*: the overproduction of fat from the *sebaceous* glands. All too often, men attempt to dry out the skin with harsh solutions, trying to remove oil. In fact, using an oil blend to treat the sebaceous glands actually slows down the skin's secretions and the essential oil moves easily into the pores to treat the skin. It is often best to treat an oily skin with an oil-based product, therefore, essential oils applied daily in a base carrier oil such as *Jojoba* will help to balance these oil secretions.

Essential oil treatments combined with a sensible diet, exercise, fresh air and regular sunlight (sunbathing, not sun*baking* which can make your skin worse) and fresh air often clear up the problem. Lymphatic flow is increased by using the oils, allowing much-needed oxygen and other nutrients to reach the skin in greater quantity.

Essential oils are *lipophilic* which means they love fat and oil. They have a direct affinity to the *sebum* in your skin and are therefore quickly absorbed into the body via the hair follicle. Their bactericide and anti-inflammatory properties are extremely useful in helping the healing process. The relaxant properties of essential oils also play their part, as stress is a precursor to increased sebum production.

There are very specific oils which act to cleanse and detoxify the skin, and others that function with the primary task of stimulating cell renewal. As acne can cause scarring, these regenerating oils are particularly beneficial.

Many men try to dry out their skin thinking that this will stop the oil production, but in fact the nerve endings in the skin register that it is dry, so it produces even *more* oil. Whereas if you apply an *oil* to the face or body to treat the acne, these same nerve endings will know that there is an ample supply of oil, and consequently slow down its production.

Stimulants and addictive foods like alcohol, coffee, tea, chocolate and refined sugar should be avoided. Smoking can aggravate acne and pimples - a fact overlooked by many young people who take up smoking only to find that their skin pays a horrible price.

MASSAGE OIL TREATMENT
FOR ACNE AND OILY SKIN

Mornings

Cypress – 1 drop		Bergamot – 1 drop
Lemon – 1 drop	or	Cypress – 1 drop
Tea Tree – 1 drop		Juniper – 1 drop

Mix with 5mls of Jojoba oil in a glass bowl.

Apply a small amount of these blended oils to the face and massage gently into the skin.

ACNE SCARRING

Mornings and Evenings

Apply *Lavender* oil neat to the skin with a cotton bud to small areas only. If treating larger areas, the essential oil must be blended into a base massage oil.

COMPRESSES

Mornings and Evenings

| Chamomile – 2 drops | Lavender – 2 drops |
| Patchouli – 2 drops | |

Add the oils to a basin of warm to hot water and agitate to disperse the oils. Drop in a clean face cloth and squeeze excess water out. Press cloth to the skin. Repeat this six times.

Shaving

If you thought you had it bad having to shave every day or so, think again. The ancient Egyptians literally hacked away their whiskers with pumice stone, and some African tribes singed off their facial hair with hot irons! Thankfully, the safety razor was invented in 1762, which made the removal of unwanted hair a tad less painful.

Still, for many men, shaving is about as much fun as going to the dentist, and sometimes just as painful. If you have coarse, fast-growing facial hair or sensitive skin, you'd probably love some tips to make this everyday task an enjoyable one. And no wonder! Shaving every day is akin to scraping sandpaper over your face, and it can sometimes injure the protective layers of the skin and cause a great deal of discomfort.

But that's just the beginning. In the hope of achieving some soothing relief and a refreshing fragrance, many men use synthetic aftershave products which are often full of harsh chemicals. On some skins, these products can cause a blotchy red rash or even small pimple-like bumps.

If you have ever experienced skin irritation after using commercial skin care and aftershave products, you should seriously consider switching completely to natural products such as essential oils. The correct oils will not only soothe the skin after shaving and give it a wonderful, fresh feeling, they'll also make you smell great, will promote a feeling of wellbeing and, when used properly, won't irritate the skin. In fact, they will even have a therapeutic effect!

If you're like most men, you probably haven't given much thought to skin care at all, let alone considered the possibility of making your own products. But think about it. It's the best way to make sure you know exactly what you're putting on your skin; it costs less, doesn't require excess packaging and no animals have suffered in the making of the product, either through testing or the use of animal by-products.

Don't worry, you don't need a degree in chemistry or a diploma in beauty therapy to make your own blends. You can learn more about the properties of each oil in Chapter 2. But for now, here are a couple of suggestions you might like to try. The after-shave splash is refreshing, antiseptic and spot-clearing and is the perfect shaving standby. And don't forget your pre-shave soak and skin regenerator listed on the previous pages.

Antiseptic After-Shave Splash
Lavender — 2 drops   Bergamot — 2 drops
Tea Tree — 2 drops
Mix into a 100ml bottle filled with water.
Take a small amount into your hands and splash it on the face.

Romance After-Shave Splash
Rosewood — 2 drops   Ylang Ylang — 2 drops
Mandarin — 2 drops
Mix into a 100ml bottle filled with water.
Take a small amount into your hands and splash it on the face.

Passion After-Shave Splash
Palmarosa — 2 drops   Jasmine — 2 drops
Black Pepper — 2 drops
Mix into a 100ml bottle filled with water.
Take a small amount into your hands and splash it on the face.

Skin Repair (Sensitivity) Blend
Lavender — 25 drops   Bergamot — 10 drops
Sandalwood — 15 drops
Mix into 100mls of Jojoba oil.
Massage a small amount into the skin in the mornings.

Tonifying Blend (For open pores)

Lemon — 10 drops	*Grapefruit — 5 drops*
Sage — 20 drops	*Cypress — 15 drops*

Mix into 100mls of Jojoba oil.

Dab onto the skin with a cotton ball.

So, gentlemen, if you're not the full-beard type, there's no need to suffer in silence. As many women who shave their legs and armpits have discovered, essential oils can help make the whole hair affair a great deal more pleasant.

First Aid

The three essentials:

Lavender is the outdoor adventurer's saviour and especially useful for campers.

- It is great for calming burns. Apply directly to the burn unless the skin is broken.
- It will alleviate the itch of mosquito bites and take the sting out of ant or other insect bites. Apply directly to the skin.
- It can be used on Stinging Nettle rash and most other rashes for that matter. Apply directly to the skin.
- It is also great for sunburn, especially when made up into a massage blend with *Jojoba* oil, or blended into an aromatic splash to pour over the area.

Tea Tree oil is a wonderful antiseptic.

- It can be used on most small infected sites. Apply directly to the infected area with a cotton bud.
- It can be dabbed on inflamed pimples. Apply neat with a cotton bud or use it as an antiseptic wash by adding 5

drops of *Tea Tree* oil to 100mls of water. Gently shake the bottle to disperse the molecules, then pour over the affected area.

Peppermint is the traveller's aid for nausea and travel sickness. It is the classic stomach remedy to settle and disperse indigestion.

• Simply remove the lid and inhale directly from the bottle or place several drops onto a handkerchief and inhale.

• A vaporiser dispersing *Peppermint* into the air is invaluable in any environment to settle and calm.

• When applying *Peppermint* to the body, blend 2 drops into 5mls of massage base oil and gently massage the blend over the chest for aromatic benefits, and over the stomach for healing benefits.

Care for the Genital Area

Essential oils can greatly assist male hygiene and sexual health. Try the following wash and massage blends.

Antibacterial Wash Blend
Bergamot — 2 drops   *Lavender — 2 drops*
Tea Tree — 2 drops

Anti-inflammatory Massage Blend
Bergamot — 10 drops   *Lavender — 25 drops*
German Chamomile — 15 drops
Add to 100mls of Jojoba oil.

Rejuvenating Massage Blend
Juniper — 10 drops   *Lavender — 25 drops*
Sandalwood — 15 drops
Add to 100mls of Jojoba oil.

4

Let it Shine

AROMATHERAPY FOR
HAIR CARE AND BALDING

"It's a funny thing hair. Just when it
seems you're destined to go bald on top.
it starts growing out your nose.
It's like the hair is still in your head,
but decides it's time to pop out for
a breather elsewhere."

Steve Martin, actor & comedian

While American actor Steve Martin makes light
of balding, for many men it's no laughing matter. Male
self-image and self-confidence can be greatly reduced by
baldness. Indeed, men seem to worry about their hair (or
lack thereof) about as much as women worry about their

weight. It's a sensitive issue, but one which can be addressed with aromatherapy.

In speaking with men at our seminars, we have discovered that they feel their hair is an important asset and certainly worthy of some attention in order to keep it.

Basically, our genetic makeup determines how much hair we lose as we age. Fortunately, the essential oils have proven quite helpful in reducing hair loss by improving the health of the scalp and the person in general. Remember, too, that the way we handle stress, shock, trauma, illness or change can influence the degree of hair loss we experience.

Several new drugs and potions have helped stimulate hair growth, and cosmetic surgery has helped many men, but these are drastic measures. The right haircut can also do wonders. The almost universal rule when dealing with thinning hair is: *less is more*. If the hair is kept shorter, it actually appears fuller. A 'Caesar' cut, like the one Kevin Costner sported in the film, *The Bodyguard*, creates a false hairline and evens out thinning patches.

We believe the first step for all men concerned about hair loss should be to work with essential oils as part of a new hair care program. Several of the essential oils can very effectively stimulate atrophied hair follicles into producing hair growth. Not only that, but the oils - unlike chemical drugs - are harmless to the body if used correctly. It's a shame the same can't be said about the drugs and potions often recommended. You may already know that the skin is the largest organ of the body and it must be nourished and cared for in order for it to function well.

Don't expect the essential oils to work miracles. They can't restore a full head of hair overnight, but they can help a great deal. It's important to realise that you'll be doing your hair a great service if you work on the whole body with the essential oils - not just your head. The circulatory and lymphatic systems should also be worked on, particularly through massage.

Essential Oils To Stimulate Hair Growth
Juniper, Rosemary, Neroli, Lavender, Geranium, Basil, Cypress, Sandalwood, Cedarwood

Use these oils singly or in a combination of three. Add three to five drops in total to a bath or massage a blend into the scalp. Warm oil treatments can be applied once a week or up to four times a week during the initial six weeks of the program.

Hair Growth Stimulation Blends
Rosemary — 20 drops	*Cedarwood — 10 drops*
Juniper — 15 drops	*Cypress — 5 drops*

Add to 100mls *Jojoba* oil and massage into the scalp night and morning. To remove oil from the hair, apply shampoo before adding water to emulsify the oil, then rise.

You can place two drops of each of the same oils into 100mls of distilled water as a final aromatic hair rinse each time you was your hair.

Hair Care

Like your skin, your hair is the outer expression of your inner health, reflecting either the balance or imbalance of the physical state you are in. Dry, oily or thinning hair can communicate the message that something is amiss internally.

If you care about your health, then it makes sense that you should make the effort to care for your hair properly. Poor health, whatever its cause, leads to hair that lacks luster and life. An Australian scientist, Kenneth Seaton, has shown that there is an incredible relationship between the hair and the immune system.

"Damage to the hair can damage immunity," says Seaton, who has spent much time studying the relationship between hair, baldness, graying and ageing.

"Similarly," he says, "damage to the immune system, and health in general, will always be indicated by a poor-looking head of hair. Striking evidence of this is that in any serious disease, hair loss is evident. Little wonder that shiny, strong, healthy hair has always indicated a healthy body."

The message is clear - do not treat your hair as if it has no role to play. Care for it just as you would your teeth or your skin. Get a good cut which suits your face shape and have regular trims. Avoid harsh detergent-based shampoos or soaps. Go for a shampoo that contains only natural ingredients and don't stick to the same shampoo and conditioner week-in, week-out.

Remember, the milder shampoos are less likely to strip the hair of its acid mantle. Conditioners should be rich in proteins. You can add essential oils to commercial products, enhancing the efficacy of the products and making them personal to you.

As an added bonus, oils can also enhance the natural colour of your hair. *Chamomile* and *Lemon* are effective in lightening blonde hair; *Sage, Rosemary* and *Sandalwood* promote lustre and shine on brunette or black hair; *Orange* and *Bergamot* enhance ginger or red hair.

Hair Blends

Utensils: 100ml glass bottle for blending, *Jojoba* massage base oil (*Jojoba* strengthens the hair follicle and shaft. Given that *Jojoba* is a fixed wax, it coats the hair and is easier to work with than an oil.)

Instructions:

Fill your empty blending bottle with *Jojoba* and add your essential oils (choose from the suggested blends below). Massage the blend into the scalp daily or weekly, depending on the severity of the condition. When removing the oil, add shampoo to the hair *before* adding water to emulsify the oil, then rinse thoroughly.

You can use your aromatic blend as a rinse or hair tonic.

Hair Tonic

Take two drops of your blended essential oils and add them to 2mls of water. Massage into the scalp and through the hair at night so the oils can do their work whilst the body is in repair.

Hair Rinse

Add a total of five drops of essential oils to 100ml blending bottle filled with warm water. Shake the bottle and pour the blend through the hair before leaving the shower in the morning.

Sensitive Scalp Blend

Lavender — 20 drops   *Bergamot — 10 drops*
Sandalwood — 20 drops

Oily Hair Blend
Bergamot — 20 drops   Sage — 13 drops
Cypress — 17 drops

Anti-Dandruff Blend
Tea Tree — 20 drops   Rosemary — 20 drops
Cedarwood — 10 drops

Damaged Hair Blend
Geranium — 10 drops   Lavender — 20 drops
Sandalwood — 20 drops

Loss of Hair Blend
Juniper — 15 drops   Rosemary — 20 drops
Cedarwood — 15 drops

5

Getting Down to Business

AROMATHERAPY IN THE OFFICE

"MEN HAVE BEEN CHAINED TO THEIR WORK
AND NEED TO FIND MORE BALANCE IN THEIR
LIVES. IT WILL BE A LIBERATING MOMENT
WHEN MEN REALISE THEY DON'T HAVE TO LIVE
UP TO SOME TOUGH AUSSIE MALE IMAGE,
THAT THE MAJORITY OF US HAVE WARM
HEARTS AND SWEET SOULS."

Richard Glover, Sydney Morning Herald columnist

THE MAJORITY OF MEN SPEND A MINIMUM OF about eight hours of every day in the work environment, perhaps even more.

Think about your home or your bedroom for a moment. You or your partner have probably made at least some, if not a lot of effort making it comfortable. If you spend a lot of time there you probably want it to be a pleasurable, inviting place to be - a sanctuary.

Well, you also spend a lot of time at work, so why not do the same for your work environment? Of course, most people don't feel the need to fill up their work space with personal possessions the way they do in their homes. But to do your job properly, you have to feel at ease in your environment and have effective tools to support you to be purposeful and productive.

Essential oils are a practical, convenient and no-fuss way to put your own personal stamp on your work space. All too often we are influenced by someone else's opinion of what we do and end up succumbing to peer group pressure. We say this because many men have told us, "My colleagues will think I've gone hippy".

We invite you to continue to create support mechanisms in your life that will diminish stress and enhance your identity. By filling your office with a specifically designed combination of oils you can set the mood of the day, lift your spirits when necessary, aid concentration, reduce stress, remain alert and create a harmonious and creative work environment. Tall orders from those small bottles perhaps, but remember, essential oils are 70 times more concentrated than the plant they come from.

To understand this, imagine the inner power that dwells within your body. It's certainly not limited to your cell structure - you are capable of producing so much more energy when it is called upon. Essential oils work in exactly the same way.

Let's say you have to make an important presentation today. You spent all night tossing and turning (which could have been alleviated with essential oils!), worrying about how it will go. Your stomach churns all morning and you can't eat. You go into the boardroom feeling less than alert and energetic. By the end of the day you've had it. The stress of the day has taken its toll and you might resort to cigarettes, alcohol or junk food for comfort.

The alternative scenario could be that you take a long, warm, relaxing aromatic bath the night before. After inhaling the relaxing vapours and letting them penetrate your skin, you're ready for a peaceful night's sleep. You wake up feeling refreshed, even though still a little nervous.

You mix a blend that will calm your nerves and vaporise it while eating breakfast and getting ready. Previously, you had studied your subject while burning a special *Total Recall Blend*, (to enhance memory retention - see the end of this chapter) which you take to work with you. Throughout the morning and just before you begin the presentation, you inhale the scent deeply from an oil-laden handkerchief, allowing all the information to come flowing easily from your memory banks. The presentation is a success and you arrive home feeling on top of the world!

You can use aromatherapy on any normal working day. On arriving at your workplace, decide upon the mood that you want to establish for the day (peaceful, mentally stimulating, creative etc.) before you sit at your desk or start your activities. Arrive five minutes earlier if you have to so you can light your vaporiser and create your aromatic blend for the day. You can also change the aromatic combinations very quickly and easily at lunch time to produce a change in the work environment for the second half of the day.

Have nearby, either in your desk drawer or briefcase, a flannel or face washer. During the day, take the flannel to the bathroom and rinse it under very hot water to saturate the cloth. Add two or three drops of essential oil and squeeze out the flannel so the excess water is removed. Then hold the flannel to your face, cupped in both hands, and inhale deeply three times. Breathe in for a count of five and out for a count of five. Do this three times. We guarantee this will contribute greatly to your day and leave you feeling energetic and balanced emotionally. Remember, by inhaling essential oils in this way, you can change the way you feel in four seconds!

If you work outdoors or are on the move, leave a few drops of oil on a handkerchief or on a cotton wool square which you can drop into a pocket to carry around with you during the day.

Office Blends

Utensils: A vaporiser, 9-hour vaporiser candles, matches, water (to place in the top of the vaporiser), your essential oil selection.

Instructions:

Add 8 drops in total of essential oil to the water in the top of your *In Essence* vaporiser. Light the candle in the base of the unit. As the water warms, the aromatic vapour will help to dissipate the oils around the room, and the heat from the candle will continue to keep the water warm. Use your vaporiser in the office or board room.

We recommended that you use one blend in the morning and change the combination in the afternoon because our sense of smell fatigues when exposed to the same smell for a period of time. Life is not a static state; habits don't happen in nature, so we need to keep the body guessing by keeping our senses aroused and awake to changes.

Refresh and Uplift
Bergamot — 3 drops   Lemongrass — 2 drops
Black Pepper — 3 drops

Stimulate and Activate the Mind
Rosemary — 3 drops   Lemon — 2 drops
Cardamon — 3 drops

Settle and Calm
Lavender — 3 drops   Neroli — 3 drops
Palmarosa — 2 drops

Promote Inspiration
Pine — 3 drops   Basil — 2 drops
Bergamot — 3 drops

Promote Productivity (Especially post-lunch)
Peppermint — 3 drops   Lemon — 3 drops
Juniper — 2 drops

Mental Focus and Clarity
Lemon — 4 drops   Rosemary — 2 drops
Black Pepper — 2 drops

Confidence and Optimism
Sandalwood — 3 drops   Orange — 3 drops
Jasmine Absolute — 2 drops

Boosting Morale
Grapefruit — 3 drops   Petitgrain — 3 drops
Frankincense — 2 drops

Invigorator Blend
Eucalyptus — 3 drops   Lemongrass — 2 drops
Sage — 3 drops

Open Communication & Creativity
Orange — 2 drops   Bergamot — 3 drops
Frankincense — 3 drops

Insomnia Blend
Lavender — 3 drops   Marjoram — 2 drops
Orange — 3 drops

Pre-Presentation Jitters Blend
Bergamot — 3 drops   Mandarin — 3 drops
Sandalwood — 2 drops

Commuting

No matter how you get to work and home again, you can use these techniques to influence your environment:

On A Handkerchief or Tissue
Lemon — 4 drops   Rosemary — 1 drop
Clary Sage — 1 drop

Inhale to keep alert and uplifted through the hustle and bustle. Also useful if you're feeling a little lethargic mid-afternoon. Take three deep breaths - counting to five as you breathe in and out.

On The Dashboard (Rub on):

Lavender – *2 drops*   *Rosewood* – *1 drop*

As the sun shines through the window, the warmth will vaporise the oils into the car. This is a great blend to soothe, calm and disperse anxiety or stress.

Air Conditioner or Heater Duct

Place an aromatic tissue which has your favourite relaxing oils over the air conditioner or heater duct so that the air which enters the car smells cleaner and fresher as you drive. Play a tape of your favourite music as you breathe in the aromatic air, and traffic jams will never be the same again!

Spray Pack

Keep this handy at work. Add 2 drops of *Bergamot* to a small (approx 100mls) spray bottle of water (must be glass). Shake well. This can be used as an aromatic skin tonic and freshener. The *Bergamot* will tonify and cleanse your skin while bringing a sense of lightness to uplift your spirit.

No matter where you work or what position you hold, you will always be able to create a space you can call your own. If you share an office, your co-workers will also benefit and you may even spark off an aromatherapy trend among your colleagues. No doubt many of them will have already used oils at home, so why not be the first to bring a point of difference to the office?

Study

There are more adults studying today than ever before. Improving ourselves has become a way of life. What usually accompanies learning is the subsequent examination. Whether you are the student, or someone you know is, there's one thing you can usually count on... not looking forward to that final test! Have you ever met anyone who likes exams? We haven't, but we've met hundreds who find them completely nerve-racking. Some people make themselves so sick over the possibility of failure that no matter how much they have studied, they forget everything as soon as they're in the examination room. It's almost as if the simple fear of forgetting everything is what *makes* them forget!

Using aromatherapy to help you study and recall the information during the exam is the closest you can get to virtually having your text books in front of you. That's how effective it is! If only *we* had known about essential oils when we were at school....

Exams are not just the bane of the school-aged, especially if you're concerned with furthering your career or self-development. Some of you are lucky enough to be gifted with great memories, and probably find exams a breeze. For the rest of us, essential oils can be powerful weapons with which to arm ourselves before going into the exam room.

Essential oils are so effective for study because they register in the brain's *limbic* system, that place where our memory is stored. Our thirty years' combined experience as therapists and feedback from other creditable aromatherapists has shown that if the pure particles of a specially-chosen essential oil penetrate your limbic system at the same time you are filling it with new information, guess what happens? The next time you smell that particular oil, the information comes flooding back. It's as simple as that! We call this *odour association*.

This method is especially effective for high school students who may have to study several unrelated subjects at the same time. A new scent can be chosen for each subject, thus eliminating any confusion and assisting the student to maintain complete focus and clarity. So if you or your children suffer from those horrible pre-exam nerves, don't despair, let aromatherapy help.

Instructions:

The following blends can be used in your vaporiser (8 drops in total). You can choose the combinations of each - we recommend blending by preference. Alternatively, you can use them in a massage blend as per the following recipes, blending into 100mls of massage base oil. If you are going to place the oils in combination onto a handkerchief to inhale, just use one drop of each.

Pre-Exam Blend
Bergamot — 20 drops   *Neroli — 15 drops*
Petitgrain — 15 drops

Study Blend
Basil — 15 drops   *Lemon — 25 drops*
Pine — 10 drops

Total Recall Blend
Rosemary – 25 drops   *Lemon – 15 drops*
Basil – 10 drops

Creativity Blend
Orange – 20 drops   *Rosemary – 15 drops*
Black Pepper – 15 drops

At Home

Simply fill your vaporiser with water, add 8 drops in total of essential oil to the water in the top of your *In Essence* vaporiser. Light the candle in the base of the unit. As the aroma disperses into the air, your mind will link the experience with the odour.

In the Exam Room

Dispense the same blend as drops of oil onto a handkerchief and inhale as you progress through your paper.

Beating Stress

For centuries humans have recognised the power of thought in our lives. William Shakespeare wrote, "There is nothing either good or bad, but thinking makes it so." Today, many people will agree that thought, the mind, is the major determinant of how our lives will go. Change your thoughts and you change your world.

Our futures are formed by the thoughts we hold most often in our minds and subsequently speak about. If we think and talk about how bad our lives are going, then chances are our lives will continue to be miserable. Conversely, if we look on the positive side of life, accept that life is not always going to be a breeze, and focus on the good things in our life, we're likely to be happier and more content.

Stress is perhaps the number one health concern of the '90s, and most of us are aware of it to some extent. Stress can be positive or negative, but we cannot avoid it. To undertake any challenge we need a certain amount of stress, that's natural. However, it becomes unhealthy when we let stress become distress.

Distress is another thing altogether. This is when our stress becomes chronic, perhaps as a result of a series of ongoing events. The result is that we lose energy and our love of life is traded for frustration and sometimes victimisation.

This is when the essential oils come into their own, uplifting our spirits and centering our emotions.

Everyone handles stress differently. Stress takes place within ourselves and must be addressed individually. It never ceases to amaze us how the essential oils can help. We really do have healing and calming substances at our very fingertips—or noses as the case may be.

With our aromatic wardrobe we can dress emotionally for every occasion. Indeed, we believe if everyone had an aromatic wardrobe and used it to contribute to the way they want to feel and think, we would have a far more effective world.

We see essential oils as our friends. They are there to service us 100 per cent of the time. All we have to do is act and initiate the responses we desire.

THE STRESS BUSTERS

Stress is a force that can strain and deform or renew and empower. The essential oils can truly help us calm our emotions, clear our minds and focus more clearly on what we wish to achieve.

Next time you feel as though you are being pushed to the brink and that you can't cope with one more crying child, one more demanding phone call, one more bill to pay, one more nerve-wracking day at the office, we invite you to inhale, bathe or massage with the aid of some stress-reducing aromas and watch your tensions slip away. We guarantee you'll be impressed with the results!

Pick me Ups

Bergamot — 4 drops   *Cedarwood — 2 drops*
Lavender — 2 drops
or
Orange — 4 drops   *Sandalwood — 2 drops*
Ylang Ylang — 2 drops
or
Bergamot — 4 drops   *Geranium — 2 drops*
Patchouli — 2 drops

Defeat Depression

When we are sad and troubled, we need a little something to uplift and make us feel better in ourselves and about ourselves.

So we can use *Ylang Ylang*, *Rose* or *Clary Sage* together, singularly or with other oils, until we feel once again in control of our emotions.

Sadly, there are currently tens of thousands of people in Australia taking tranquillisers. Many of these people will become addicted to their medication and function poorly without them. Some remain in a half-drugged, half-alive state for years.

Breathing in the aromas of nature makes us feel more beautiful and tranquil and helps us to engage our inner strength to transform the worries of the day. We truly believe that the essences are one of God's gifts to us, and by inhaling their beauty they help us to experience the joys of life once again.

Depression Buster Massage Blends

Soothing Nervous Butterflies
Bergamot — 22 drops   Basil — 9 drops
Lavender — 19 drops
In 100mls of massage base oil.

For Chronic Anxiety
Lavender — 22 drops   Cedarwood — 19 drops
Lemongrass — 9 drops

For Acute Anxiety
Lavender — 22 drops   Geranium — 9 drops
Sandalwood — 19 drops
In 100mls of massage base oil.

These formulas can be modified to create smaller massage blends, ie five drops of essential oil into 10mls of massage base oil. Remember always the 1:2 ratio. For every drop of essential oil, add 2mls of massage base oil.

Making your Own formulas to Beat Stress

As you become more proficient with the essential oils, you can make your own blends to treat all types of ailments and emotional conditions. For stress-related conditions, the oils can be used singly or in a combination of three. It helps to understand what oils act as stimulants, and what oils act as sedatives or relaxants.

STIMULANTS

Basil, Clary Sage, Cypress, Eucalyptus, Fennel, Geranium, Juniper, Lemon, Lemongrass, Neroli, Peppermint, Pine, Rose, Rosemary, Sage, Tea Tree, Thyme, Black Pepper, Cardamon, Ginger, Grapefruit, Lime, Palmarosa, Petitgrain.

SEDATIVES/RELAXANTS

Chamomile Roman, Chamomile German, Basil, Cedarwood Frankincense, Lavender, Geranium, Marjoram, Myrrh, Neroli, Orange, Patchouli, Rose, Sandalwood, Vetiver, Ylang Ylang, Jasmine Absolute, Mandarin, Rosewood, Cardamon, Petitgrain.

You will notice that some oils appear in both lists. This is because of the phenomenon called "adoptogens"––these are essential oils which act as natural balancers and instigate a reaction in the body that is appropriate to achieve a state of 'homeostasis' or balance.

6

Animal Magnetism

AROMATHERAPY IN THE
BEDROOM AND BATHROOM

"I THINK PROBABLY LOVE IS BEING AT YOUR
FULLEST, AND AT YOUR FULLEST MOMENT
BEING WILLING TO GIVE THAT OVER TO
SOMEONE ELSE OR TO SOME OTHER THING."

Robert Redford, actor

FROM TIME IMMEMORIAL ESSENTIAL OILS HAVE been used to
seduce the senses into a magical euphoria, to lull the mind into
a deep sense of relaxation or to arouse the body awareness.
Let's explore how we can use these qualities today.

One of the great attributes of essential oils is their ability
to stimulate and re-charge our physical and mental states.
We can use aromatics to alter our moods and emotions. The
essences work on our physiology, uplifting our spirits and

helping us to rise above the logical or linear thinking that can sometimes effect our emotional wellbeing or interfere with our being connected to our feelings.

Aromatic oils can be used very effectively to create a mood for intimacy and lovemaking. When aroma and romance come together we create "aromatic romance" and this really is one of the fun things about essential oils.

Imagine returning home after an intimate dinner for two and being greeted with the sensually-stimulating aroma of your romance blend of *Patchouli, Ylang Ylang* and *Orange* rising from your vaporiser.

With lashings of essential oil and a little imagination, you can add a wonderful new dimension to your love life. Some of our clients have said our aromatic romance suggestions have helped them rekindle passion in their relationship. Certainly, the oils have been used very effectively to reactivate diminished sex drives in both males and females.

The alluring oils will help you to respond positively to your partner, and if you are both contributing to a deep-seated love and respect for one another, the essential oils will truly work wonders.

Certain essential oils have "heady", euphoric characteristics, so why not take your favourite and imbue your bedroom? Create an aromatic setting that will sweep you and your partner into a mood of scentual awareness and sexual excitement.

Jasmine, Rose, Patchouli, Orange, Ylang Ylang and *Palmarosa* are ideal for bedrooms and seduction. *Rose* is arguably the favourite perfume of all time, and is an integral ingredient in many modern-day perfumes. One drop of oil on a piece of cotton wool, slipped under the pillow slip or between the sheets can work wonders.

A word to the wise. Like anything else in life, there is no magic potion that will make your love life work for you. We believe that it is not just the properties of essential oils that work in this area. Even more importantly, it is the *intention* behind the blend. If you use these blends with an expectation of another to perform - guess what? The bigger the expectation, the bigger the disappointment.

A man we will call John once attended a weekend workshop with us and couldn't wait to get home on the Saturday evening to try out *Ylang Ylang* on his wife. The following morning he arrived with a look of disappointment. He told us that he had gone home that evening, "ran the bath like you told me; threw in some *Ylang Ylang* and told the Missus to get in. When she got out, nothing!" he said with dismay.

We told him that had he lit a candle in the bathroom to set the mood, washed and bathed himself in preparation for lovemaking or invited her to participate with him in the bath, he might have had the result he was after.

To achieve a goal, you must have a plan of action and have your own actions be congruent with the outcome you are wanting. Don't expect the oils to do all the wooing for you! Seduction is a gentle and skilled art form - and practice makes perfect!

Aphrodisiacs

Certain essential oils have long been praised for their aphrodisiac qualities. One of the reasons they work so fast and effectively is because they act directly on that part of the brain which governs our hormones and is also responsible for sexual behaviour and response.

In a less direct way, other essences possess the ability to spark fatigued reproductive glands into action, and so work to revive a waning interest in sex. Study the sensuality blends in our book *Aromatherapy for Lovers and Dreamers* for some extra tips. Give your love life the inspiration and vitality it deserves. Being fully self-expressed in all areas of your life continues to contribute to your health and wellbeing. To keep the relationship healthy and vital, talk to your partner and ask if they are feeling fulfilled. Explore aromatic blends together to open communication.

Massage

Something that proves extreamly pleasurable and seductive is a good body massage performed by strong, loving hands, but many people refrain from using this simple technique because they don't know how to go about it. Here are some tips to start you massaging today.

The right essential oil blend, loving care and sensitivity, a little time and energy, and a good pair of hands is all you need to begin practising massage. Set the scene in advance by warming the room, putting on some comfortable clothes and focusing your energy on what you're about to do.

There is no hard and fast rule as to what areas of the body should be massaged first or last, but many experienced massage therapists follow a basic sequence of back, shoulders and neck, back of legs, arms and hands, front of legs, front of torso, face and scalp. They usually work in strokes moving toward the lymph nodes.

If you're performing the massage purely for relaxation purposes, avoid stimulating the nipple and genital areas as much as possible. Your partner must know the type of massage you are about to give so they can respond appropriately. Apply discipline to a relaxation massage to build trust in your partner by not violating this sacred space.

Gliding Strokes
Gentle, rhythmic hand strokes over all parts of the body. Just let your hands float over the skin without applying too much pressure. You can try moving your hands in broad circles - a good stroke for spreading the oil evenly over the body.

Medium-Depth Strokes
Following on from the gliding strokes, you can now start to work more deeply on the large muscle masses, using kneading, pushing and pulling strokes. Keep the rhythm constant and flowing.

Deep Tissue Strokes - Deep and focused, these friction movements use the thumbs, fingertips or heels of hands to reach right down into the tissue to where more hidden tensions may lie.

Percussion Strokes
Stimulating rather than relaxing, percussion strokes are performed repeatedly with alternating hands. Hacking, cupping and pummeling with your fists or hands all have a regenerating effect. Remember to be careful when pummelling, especially if you tend to be heavy-handed. Let your partner's level of enjoyment be your best guide.

Feathering

This is a brief, delicate stroke which brushes over the surface of the skin. It is mainly used to break contact gently.

MASSAGE BLENDS

The basic rule for massage blends is a 2-1 ratio. That is, for every 2mls of massage base oil you will need approx 1 drop of essential oil. For example, add three - five drops of essential oil in total to every 10mls of *Sweet Almond* oil for a general massage. When using several essential oils in your blend you have the choice to proportion the drops accordingly so that they add up to the total number of drops required.

Keep a small mixing bowl handy for blending and always use glass containers. The following blends should be placed into 20mls of massage base oil, so you would add 10 drops of essential oil to make the correct prescriptive blend. When doing a full body massage, we recommend you begin with 20mls of massage base oil.

Relaxation Blend
Bergamot — 3 drops   Cedarwood — 4 drops
Neroli — 3 drops
Into 20mls of massage base oil.

Magic Moment Blend
Orange — 2 drops   Rose — 4 drops
Sandalwood — 4 drops
Into 20mls of massage base oil.

Rejuvenation Blend
Frankincense — 4 drops   Neroli — 4 drops

Lavender — 2 drops
Into 20mls of massage base oil.

Seduction Blend
Ylang Ylang — 4 drops   *Clary Sage — 2 drops*
Jasmine Absolute — 4 drops
Into 20mls of massage base oil.

Restoration Blend
Lemon — 2 drops   *Rosemary — 2 drops*
Black Pepper — 2 drops   *Lavender — 4 drops*
Into 20mls of massage base oil.

Stamina Blend
Lemongrass — 2 drops   *Myrrh — 2 drops*
Sandalwood — 6 drops
Into 20mls of massage base oil.

Choosing blends together with your partner can be a nurturing, bonding experience. Our book *Aromatherapy for Lovers and Dreamers* explains how to do this. Odour association techniques work well to reconnect you with your loved one, to stir your feelings and arouse your body. Having anchored your lovemaking to a particular blend or oil, you will be able to reactivate that feeling at any time.

An important tip - don't go wearing your lovemaking blend to work - your productivity will be at an all-time low as your mind floats off to be with your lover!

Bathing

In ancient times, priests would cleanse and anoint themselves daily as an act of dedication to pure thoughts and ideals.

Local lakes served as outdoor spas. Greeks introduced bathing for inner and outer therapy while the Romans brought bathing to the height of total personal pampering. Public baths became luxurious spas for cleansing, scenting and socialising. Add this quality of richness and rejuvenation to your daily program to enhance the quality of your sensory experiences and heighten your state of bliss.

If you're feeling low and could do with an added perk, try this "cell-renewal" bath as follows:

Step 1.

Warm the bathroom environment and fill your bath with warm to hot water. Have towels and robe ready.

Step 2.

Prepare your signature blend of oil into a medium-sized ceramic vessel. Make sure you are seated in a comfortable position.

Step 3.

Smooth the oil over your skin lavishly, from the toes to the upper chest area. Take a body brush and dip into your blend.

Step 4.

Begin with small circular movements over the hands, arms, shoulders, chest area, abdomen, toward the pelvis and buttocks, down the legs and embrace the feet.

Step 5.

Once the entire body has been covered you are ready to immerse yourself into your bath. Soak for 10-15 minutes in warm water.

Step 6.

Leave the water and pat the skin dry. Your body will feel alive and your senses aroused. Robe yourself to keep warm.

THE AROMATIC BATH

Bathing can also be shared as an erotic experience with your lover. Choose a blend of romantic essential oils or a combination to relax and revitalise.

Bathing is truly an art form. You can enhance the mood with candles as your only source of lighting. Light your vaporiser and enhance further the aromatic water.

If you have a partner, seat yourself at one end and your partner at the other. You can massage each other's feet while chatting or simply enjoy each other in silence.

Make sure you have a flannel each and a small rolled-up towel to support your necks if you intend staying in the bath for a while. Lean back and enjoy!

A good technique we recommend is to start with six lit candles. Wring out the flannel and place it over your face. Take in some nice deep breaths to heighten relaxation. Press the warm flannel to your face about five times. As you relax, blow out a candle––the light change further enhances relaxation. Blow out all the candles over the duration of your bath, except one which should remain the only source of light.

You can increase your sensual awareness by taking a small amount of massage oil (pre-blended for the occasion) and massage each other when you are down to your last candle. This can turn the occasion into a very seductive bath. Choose oils that enhance intimacy.

Seductive Bath Combination No 1
Ylang Ylang — 1 drop   Orange — 3 drops
Patchouli — 1 drop

Seductive Bath Combination No 2
Sandalwood — 3 drops   Lavender — 1 drop
Ylang Ylang — 1 drop

Alternatively, you can make up a masculine combination:

Frankincense — 1 drop   Bergamot — 2 drops
Sandalwood — 2 drops

The best way to use essential oils for an aromatic bath is to add them drop by drop once the bath is fully drawn. Make sure you are ready to climb in and that the doors and windows are closed so that you can take in the full healing benefits. Here are two of our favourite relaxation bath combinations for you to try. Of course, once you begin using the essential oils on a regular basis, you will soon develop your own blends.

Relaxation Bath No 1
Geranium — 1 drop   Lavender — 2 drops
Chamomile (R) — 2 drops

Relaxation Bath No 2
Bergamot — 2 drops   Basil — 1 drop
Cedarwood — 2 drops

7

Breakfast of Champions

AROMATHERAPY FOR
SPORT AND FITNESS

"I don't really think too much about
what I'll be doing for the rest of
my life. Thinking about something is a
lot more frightening than doing it.
I've always been a doer, so I just
go ahead and do it."

Kareem Abdul-Jabbar, NBA champion

Statistics show that more men stay involved with sports
after they leave school than women (not including the type
of involvement that includes relaxing with a beer in front of
the television sports shows every weekend).

For many men, actually playing sport is a way of life:
training, match days, presentations, post-match social

activities, the list goes on. For the most part, that time is enjoyable, the spirits are lifted, there is an air of healthy competition and winning or playing a good game can often bring strong feelings of elation.

Aromatherapy can help bring those wonderful, uplifting feelings back into everyday life. In fact, essential oils have a very powerful effect when used in combination with sport. For example, placing one drop of your chosen essential oil onto a wristband before playing a tennis match can have an astounding effect on the emotions.

Inhale deeply from the wristband immediately after you've played a great shot. Psychologically, the nervous system anchors to that experience, associating the feelings brought on by the great shot with the aroma. Later, when that same oil is inhaled in any situation where you're needing confidence, you can reconnect with that powerful experience of achievement.

Whatever your sport, essential oils can help create the mood and state of mind needed to perform at your peak. *Golfers* can use oils to bring about relaxation, focus and clarity; *ball players* can use the oils to stimulate and uplift them before a game; *long distance runners* can use oils to invigorate and refresh them along the way. And when it's all over, a warm bath in essential oils is a great post-game wind-down which can also help soothe sore, tired muscles.

The numerous first-aid qualities of essential oils can also come in handy for sportsmen and athletes. Wounds, abrasions, bruises, cuts and other injuries sustained during sport can be treated with essential oils. They can also help a great deal with pre-game nerves or other ailments that could impair performance such as headaches, blocked noses or sinus problems.

One particular man we knew who was working out in the gym regularly reached a point in his program where he simply couldn't seem to extend himself. He was bench pressing 100lbs and realised that it was the fear of going beyond this that held him back. On the next visit to the gym he used *Frankincense* (to release fear) on his gloves and inhaled deeply as he held the bar in his hands. He celebrated later, having pushed 120lbs for the first time. He continued to use *Frankincense* when he trained as a powerful anchor to his success.

Sports Blends

Remember, the most effective and beneficial way to use essential oils is to massage them into the body. The more area covered the greater the result. We suggest you massage these blends into your body for special results.

Recovery Blend
Eucalyptus — 20 drops   *Juniper* — 20 drops
Lemongrass — 10 drops
Into 100mls of massage base oil.
or
Eucalyptus — 20 drops   *Petitgrain* — 10 drops
Black Pepper — 20 drops
Into 100mls of massage base oil.

Marathon Blend
Myrrh — 5 drops   *Petitgrain* — 15 drops
Juniper — 10 drops   *Eucalyptus* — 20 drops
Into 100mls of massage base oil.

Athletic Blend

Peppermint — 5 drops   *Rosemary — 15 drops*
Eucalyptus — 30 drops
Into 100mls of massage base oil.

Weightlifting Blend

Frankincense — 20 drops   *Ginger — 10 drops*
Juniper — 10 drops   *Myrrh — 10 drops*
Into 100mls of massage base oil.

Anti-Arthritic Blend

Eucalyptus — 10 drops   *Lavender — 10 drops*
Frankincense — 10 drops   *Juniper — 20 drops*
Into 100mls of massage base oil.

Allergies and Hay Fever Relief Blend

Lavender — 27 drops   *Geranium — 13 drops*
German Chamomile — 10 drops
Use as a massage blend in 100mls of Jojoba and Sweet Almond oil combined.

This blend can also be used as an inhalation: Put 2 drops of each oil into a bowl of very hot water. Place your head over the bowl and cover with a towel. Inhale for up to 10 minutes.

Competition

Grapefruit — 1 drop   *Basil — 1 drop*
Rosemary — 1 drop

Inhale this combination from a wrist band to activate and energise (place 1 drop of each onto the top of your wrist band and allow it to penetrate the cloth for several minutes before wearing the band) or blend it into a massage base oil and rub it on the body in the proportions listed. Use the two-to-one ratio to create your own proportions for single-use applications.

Energiser
Eucalyptus — 15 drops   Sage — 20 drops
Mandarin — 15 drops
Into 100mls of massage base oil.

Endurance
Cardamon — 10 drops   Rosemary — 20 drops
Sandalwood — 20 drops
Into 100mls of massage base oil.

Muscle Tonic
Eucalyptus — 20 drops   Rosemary — 20 drops
Lemongrass — 10 drops
Into 100mls of massage base oil.

Tennis Elbow
Eucalyptus — 25 drops   Juniper — 15 drops
Lemongrass — 10 drops
Into 100mls of massage base oil.

Locker Room Blend (Pre-match)
Thyme — 10 drops   Lime — 15 drops
Eucalyptus — 25 drops
Into 100mls of massage base oil.

Nervous Butterflies
Bergamot — 23 drops   Basil — 10 drops
Black Pepper — 17 drops
Into 100mls of massage base oil.

Asthma/Sinusitis
Lavender — 2 drops   Marjoram — 2 drops
Eucalyptus — 2 drops

Dispense into a bowl of very hot water. Place your head over the bowl and cover both with a towel. Alternatively, dispense onto a handkerchief and inhale throughout the day.

Abrasions and Cuts
Lavender — 2 drops   Tea Tree — 3 drops
Patchouli — 3 drops
Into 100mls of distilled water.

It is important to keep skin clean and bacteria-free when it is injured. Place the blend into a glass bottle. Shake it vigorously to dispense the molecules. Swab the area with the aromatic water on a cotton wool ball.

Athlete's Foot (Anti -Fungal Swab):
Lavender — 1 drop   Tea Tree — 1 drop
Thyme — 1 drop

Drop onto a cotton bud and dab on the skin.

Bruises (Soothing Swab):
Lavender — 1 drop   Cypress — 1 drop
Juniper — 1 drop

Dampen a cotton wool square with water, dispense these drops onto the square and smooth it over the bruise. Alternatively, make up a blend in 5mls *Jojoba* oil and lightly massage it into the bruised area.

Cough Relief Blend
Basil — 10 drops   *Pine — 15 drops*
Eucalyptus — 25 drops
Into 100mls of massage base oil.

Massage the chest and upper back twice daily.

Breathe Easy Handkerchief
Eucalyptus — 2 drops   *Peppermint — 2 drops*
Pine — 2 drops

Dispense each of these drops into the centre of a clean handkerchief. Use as an inhalation throughout the day. We recommend that you don't use this handkerchief to blow your nose in, as the essential oils in this concentration are too strong for the skin.

Odour Eater Foot Powder
Sage — 2 drops   *Cypress — 1 drop*
1 tablespoon of baking powder

Place the baking powder into a bag, add your essential oils and shake well. Help the powder to dry and separate by pressing over the bag. Dust the feet with the powder and sprinkle it into your shoes. (Add *Tea Tree* oil if you are suffering from Athlete's Foot).

Odour Eater Foot Bath
Sage — 6 drops

Place drops into a warm foot bath (preferably a stainless steel bowl). Relaxing the soles of the feet can bring immediate relief to many discomfort zones in the body.

Gastritis Massage Blend
Basil — 15 drops   *Fennel — 25 drops*
German Chamomile — 10 drops
Into 100mls of massage base oil.

Headache Clear Head Inhalation
Lavender — 2 drops   *Orange — 2 drops*
Basil — 1 drop   *Palmarosa — 1 drop*

Add these drops into your vaporiser or dispense one drop of each oil into a handkerchief and inhale.

Chronic Headache Inhalation
Rose — 1 drop   *Rosemary — 1 drop*
Basil — 3 drops   *Orange — 1 drop*

Blend and inhale from a vaporiser or from a handkerchief.

Wounds *(Antiseptic Wash)*:
Tea Tree — 5 drops   *Lavender — 2 drops*
Rosewood — 2 drops
100ml bottle filled with filtered water

Apply directly to the wound as a wash. If the skin is unbroken you can bathe the wound with soaked cotton wool.

8

Taking Time Out

AROMATHERAPY FOR
REST AND RELAXATION

"I'VE FINALLY COME TO UNDERSTAND THAT
THERE IS NO SUCCESS OR FAILURE; IT'S ABOUT
FEELING YOUR RELATIONSHIP - AND PRIMARILY
YOUR RELATIONSHIP TO YOURSELF. THE MORE I
HAVE ALLOWED MYSELF TO FEEL MY LIFE, THE
STRONGER MY CONNECTION TO THE EARTH."

Kenny Loggins, Grammy Award-winning singer

NOW WE COME TO THE AREA WHERE ESSENTIAL oils really
come into their own - relaxation. Throughout our years
of professional aromatherapy, we have always been amazed
at how many people find it so difficult to relax. With the
pressures of modern-day living, taking a few deep breaths is
simply not enough to relieve stress.

However, when combined with essential oils, deep breathing becomes a different experience altogether. Breathing is central to life, and breathing exercises can revitalise and recharge your body. Oxygenating the body and learning to breathe deeply will contribute to a more relaxed body, a calmer state of mind and sound sleep - all good reasons to begin deep breathing today!

To maximise the uptake of oxygen into your body and increase your lung capacity, we recommend the following exercise for ten minutes, three times daily:

Oxygenation Blends

Using the following blends, try this breathing technique while directly breathing in the vapours.

Inhale and exhale through the nose. Close your eyes and inhale. In your mind's eye, take your breath into the abdominal area, expanding the abdominal cavity on the inhale, and contracting it on the exhale. In this way you will actually be exercising the movement of the diaphragm.

Breathing pattern:
1. Inhale for the count of four.
2. Hold for the count of sixteen.
3. Exhale for the count of eight.

This rhythmic breathing will expand your lungs, increase your oxygen uptake potential and energise. You will notice the difference in your day after doing this breathing, particularly if you are feeling lethargic.

If you discipline yourself to take these moments of reprieve regularly from a hectic schedule, this simple exercise will break up your day and alleviate stress.

The following blends will promote improved oxygenation and respiration in your body:

Eucalyptus — *3 drops*   *Tea Tree* — *2 drops*
Cedarwood — *3 drops*

Combine these essential oils to use in your vaporiser.

or

Peppermint — *3 drops*   *Lemon* — *3 drops*
Eucalyptus — *2 drops*

Combine these essential oils to use in your vaporiser.

or

Thyme — *2 drops*   *Tea Tree* — *2 drops*
Lemon — *4 drops*

Combine these essential oils to use in your vaporiser.

Experience these combinations in your vaporiser while practising breathing exercises or simply focusing on deepening and slowing your breathing.

Meditation

Just as regular physical exercise plays an important part in our lifestyle, so too does emotional poise. One of the best ways to still the mind and become balanced and centred is through meditation. In conjunction with the appropriate oils, meditation is also a most powerful anti-stress, anti-depression therapy.

We both know from experience that maintaining a state of calm and poise at work takes practise in our everyday life outside of the office environment. It's a tall order to expect this poise on demand in your everyday life, but when you practise an exercise often enough, the patterning will become a normal part of your day.

We both meditate on a daily basis. It is best to meditate upon awakening and again in the early evening. This helps you to maintain your calm emotional state throughout the day and night.

Many people mistakenly believe that meditation is only for 'alternative types', but nothing could be further from the truth. More and more people, from children to grandparents, housewives to company executives, are discovering the wonders of meditation and the joyous feelings of calm and control that come with it.

For most, meditating regularly requires a certain amount of discipline, and to begin with, the benefits can be quite subtle. Take note of the subtleties.

Meditation enables us to be aware of every part of our body. This statement may sound a little strange, but for centuries humans have recognised a struggle between heart and mind. This struggle often leaves people distressed and confused. Meditation provides an equilibrium. Meditation centres a person. When you live your life in the present, life becomes less of a struggle and you find yourself swimming contentedly upstream. On a less profound level, meditation also brings a certain calm to that neverending stream of thoughts.

Every minute of every day can be taken up with mind chatter. We have around sixty thousand thoughts each day: that's a lot of mental activity. Wouldn't it be wonderful then if we could casually observe our thoughts from afar rather than actively participate in them, where we let ourselves get caught up in unnecessary emotion, worry and concern. With meditation this is possible.

Meditation has been described as 'the mind coming to rest in the heart'. It's from this place within that we can witness our thoughts and emotions from a different perspective. Instead of pursuing each thought, we simply become aware of its flow. That is, each thought forms and dissolves again, ebbs and flows, into the consciousness from which it arose.

Meditation enables you to live the moment much like a young child does. Watching a child engaged in life can remind us of the magic of living life moment by moment. As adults we sometimes feel the need to plan and *do* rather than simply 'be'. Children are such wonderful role models, reminding us of what's possible. Through meditation we can embrace the child within and enter the playground of life.

There are many different ways to meditate. As aromatherapists and lifestyle advisers, we suggest you explore the different methods, decide which technique feels best for you, and seek out professional training if you feel it is necessary. We personally use the Primordial Sound Meditation technique, taught to us by Dr. Deepak Chopra. It's a wonderful technique and we highly recommend it. Following is a brief introduction to it.

Primordial Sound Meditation

Primordial Sound Meditation (PSM) originates in India and has been used for thousands of years. Dr Deepak Chopra recently re-introduced this ancient technique into the West. It does not relate to activity of the mind, its aim is to get to the level of the spirit—or firstly, to the level of the individual soul which is part of the same continuum.

PSM is said to help you get in touch with your own essential nature. It is a technique that allows us to take our awareness from the level of activity to a level of silence within.

Sound is used to enter this state of silence, and PSM is based on a person's individual mantra. The mantra given to you is based on the sound that was predominating in the universe when you were born. The technique originates in India and has been used for thousands of years.

According to Deepak, old sages recorded the sounds and then employed the process of Vedic mathematics to actually calculate a person's individual sound. It was quite an in-depth process that took many hours to calculate. Today, thanks to modern technology and computers, a person's individual mantra can be determined in minutes.

The mantra given corresponds to the time when an individual was coming through from a non-local awareness into a localised awareness. They were coming from the 'gap'; that is, the gap between consciousness and matter. Thus, the mantra does not take you back to the moment of your birth, it takes you back to that level of awareness where you can access universal consciousness rather than localised consciousness.

According to Deepak, by going to your essential state, which is pure unbounded consciousness, you go from a level of physical reality to the level of mental activity beyond the ego to the soul, and you find out you are universal consciousness.

Once you have your mantra and are practising PSM the way you have been taught you may find other mental activity going on at the same time. You'll probably find your attention going back and forth between the mantra and other thoughts. The idea is not to push the thoughts out: anytime you become aware that the thoughts are dominating, gently shift back to the mantra. As you proceed you'll find the thoughts will get fainter and fainter, then suddenly there comes a time when the mantra disappears altogether and so do the thoughts. According to Deepak you are now in the gap and in touch with your essential nature.

Start Meditating Now

Meditating effectively takes practise, but you can try this simple technique right now to begin.

Sit quietly on the floor in a comfortable position, making sure your spine is straight. Use a wall for support if your spine isn't used to sitting straight. Close your eyes and concentrate on your breathing. Be aware of the breath entering and leaving your nostrils and allow all thoughts to gently pass from your mind. You can help still your mind by repeating a mantra (a positive word which means something to you), or by focusing on some relaxing music or a candle. Don't try to stop thoughts occurring. Simply observe them and let them go, always returning to that still state.

Keep your mind as still as possible for at least twenty minutes each day for effective results.

There are many excellent meditation techniques available, and however you learn to meditate, you can be sure that improved health is one of the positive side-effects you will experience. Meditation helps you relax, throw off disease and approach life with a happier, more peaceful attitude.

Meditation Blends

Add to your vaporiser and place it in the room in which you meditate.

Myrrh — 2 drops	*Bergamot — 4 drops*
Frankincense — 2 drops	

or

Sandalwood — 3 drops	*Palmarosa — 3 drops*
Frankincense — 2 drops	

or

Neroli — 3 drops	*Vetiver — 3 drops*
Chamomile (Roman) — 2 drops	

or

Black Pepper — 3 drops	*Bergamot — 3 drops*
Sandalwood — 2 drops	

Sensuous Breathing

Breathing is an important part of any meditation session. As part of your practice, you may like to try this uplifting sensuous breathing exercise.

Lie on the floor on your back and relax as much as you can, letting your body "melt away" into the floor, allowing your arms and legs to flop. Close your eyes and feel your body against the floor, paying special attention to any tension points in any part of your body. Just be aware.

Now focus inside your body and ask yourself where you feel any sensation in your muscles because of your breathing into that spot. Imagine you can exhale through that part of the body and as you do experience the breath relaxing sore muscles as it filters through them.

Now that you are relaxed, you can experiment with the beautiful movements that are part of natural free breathing. When you breathe in, feel your pelvis tip back gently so there is a slight arch to your back while your abdomen and chest rise, ribs and back expand, and chin tilts forward. Then, when you exhale, your pelvis moves down again so your spine almost touches the floor, your back contracts, and your chin and head move back again exposing the front of your neck a bit more. This natural movement is a wave-like motion that flows without hesitation from each in-breath to its following out-breath and so on. Practise. Exaggerate the tiny movements at first until you get the feel of it, then it will flow naturally.

This is a wonderful ritual to do outdoors.

Epilogue

Well gentlemen, you seem to have escaped the attentions of the cosmetics industry for the last 100 years or so, but not any more! There has been a worldwide shift in beliefs about what constitutes appropriate masculine or feminine behaviour, and for men, grooming is no longer a dirty word.

Actually, until the Victorian era, it was men who were more active in physical beautification than women. To the modern male, it may be hard to believe that the ancient Egyptians and Romans rivalled women in their use of cosmetics. Even today amongst tribes in Africa, South America and New Guinea, the male decorative process is elaborate and flamboyant.

While this is not yet the case in Western society, it's not far off. Men are streaming into beauty salons all over the world. These men know that a little pampering can do wonders for the body and soul and they are rising above the macho stereotypes and learning to become their own person.

The world of aromatherapy is not about superficial beautification. Essential oils are used to arouse our senses, to stir our inner connection to nature and ourselves and to transform the chemistry of our bodies. The world is changing. No longer is it enough for you to simply look good, because you know that ultimately, if you *feel* good, you will *look* good.

In this information and technological age, we humans are crying out for more love, more heart, more communication, and we are selling out in personal growth areas - mostly in our private lives.

You can make your life more balanced and wholistic in all spheres by having more of the things you love and that are important to you in every aspect of your life. Take your vaporiser to work, an aromatic wristband to the gym, massage your mum's hands or a loved one's body or experience a loving massage yourself. Take time to rediscover your own self worth; elevate your self-esteem by giving these gifts to yourself first and topping up the well that may have run dry - then go out and contribute your magic to others!

Bibliography

Literature that we have scanned over the years helped us considerably in the compilation of this book.

We extend our thanks and appreciation to the authors of these books and journals.

Aromatherapy

The Sense of Smell, Olfaction, Report by Dr Lewis Thomas, Chancellor of Memorial Sloan Kettering Cancer Centre, New York, and Chairman of Monell Chemical Senses Centre, Philadelphia.

The Book Of Perfumes by Eugene Rimmel.

The Fragrant Pharmacy by Valerie Ann Worwood (Macmillan, London).

Aromatherapy For Women by Maggie Tisserand (Thorsons).

Using Essential Oils For Health and Beauty by Daniele Ryman (Century).

Scents and Sensuality by Judith White and Karen Downes (Nacson & Sons).

Aromatherapy – Therapy or Placebo by Arch Minchin, PhD, & Peter Young, PhD, University of Wisconsin, USA (1987).

The Book Of Massage by Lucinda Lidell with Sara Thomas, Carola Beresford Cooke and Anthony Porter (Ebury Press).

The Family Book Of Homeopathy by Dr Andrew Lockie (Penguin Books Australia).

Making the Right Choice

For effective therapeutic use, it is vital that only pure essential oils are used in aromatherapy. Do not fall into the trap of buying cheaper, impure oils. Often they do not work effectively on a therapeutic level and there may be bodily reactions to the additives.

Unscrupulous suppliers will sometimes dilute a pure essential oil in a massage base oil and pass it off as pure natural essence. For this reason, it is advisable that you purchase your oils from a reputable company.

Take Good Care

Not all plants and plant products are beneficial to health. Some are poisonous and dangerous. The authors encourage you to follow the guidelines in this book.

The material in this book is not meant to take the place of diagnosis and treatment by a qualified medical practitioner. The authors' recommendations in this book are based on their own experiences and their vast research. However, a small number of people may react indifferently to certain oils due to biochemical individuality. For this reason, the authors make no guarantees as to the effects of their use and no liability will be accepted.

Index

About the Authors

Judith White and Karen Downes are experienced Aromatherpists, health, beauty and lifestyle educators. They have both studied holistic aromatherapy in Europe the recognized centre of knowledge in this field. They have taught Aromatherapy to Doctors, Nurses, Natural Therapists, Beauty Therapists and run workshops and seminars lecturing to tens of thousands of people around the world, providing these people with the tools to transform their lives.

Their seminars and workshops were fun, practical and inspiring, giving participants many new perceptions and life skills. Today Judith resides in Australia and Karen in England and after more than two decades, they continue to uphold and share the daily self nurturing practices through the daily use of pure essential oils.

Their message is simple "You can magnify your health beauty and wellness through simple, daily, self nurturing practices infused with the power of aromatherapy "

For more information:

Contact Judith White on Judith@australianorganicbrands.com
And
Contact Karen Downes on .... karenleedownes@hotmail.com

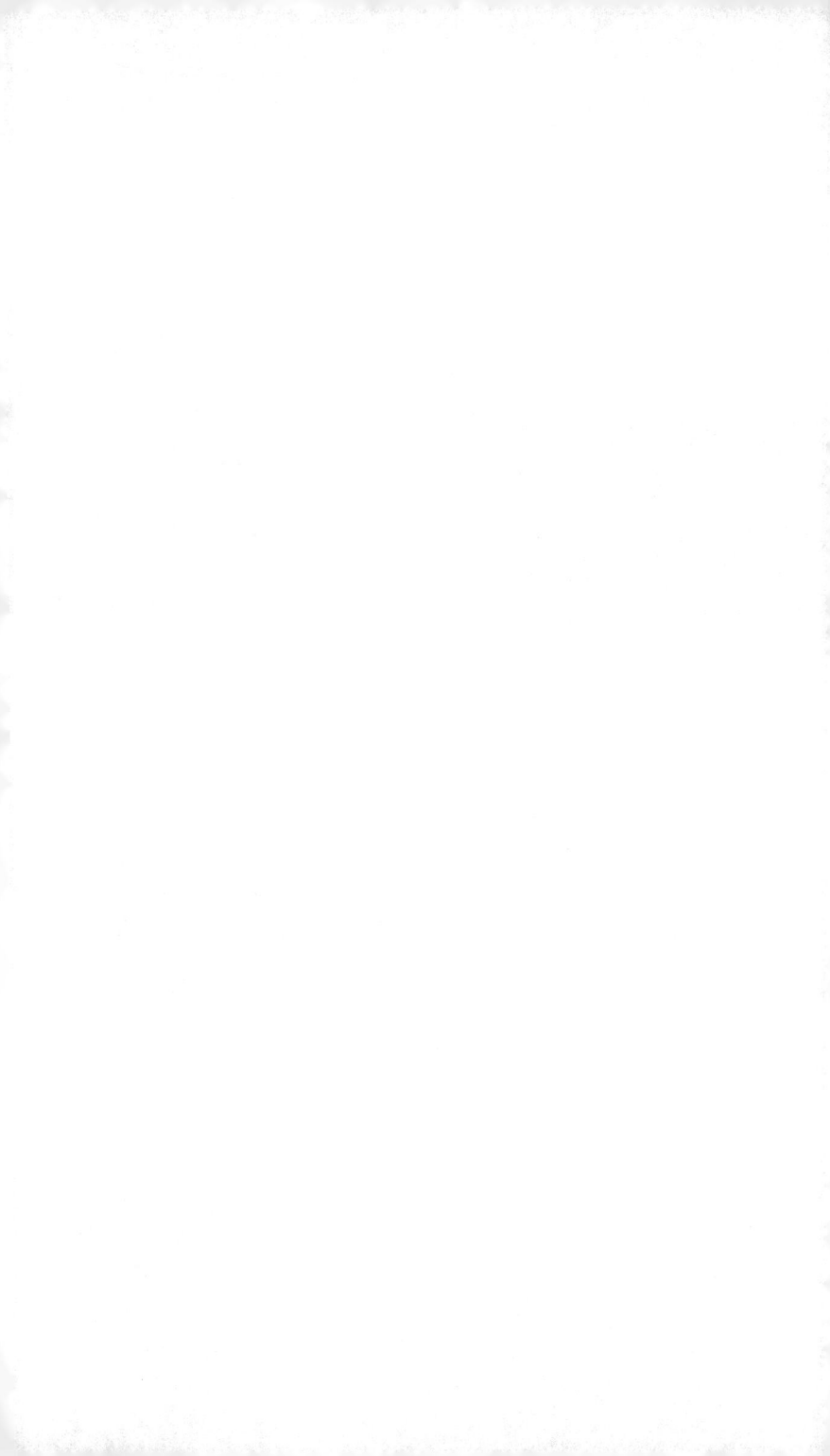